Drug Nation

Drug Nation
Patterns, problems, panics, and policies

Martin Plant

Roy Robertson

Moira Plant

Patrick Miller

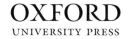
OXFORD
UNIVERSITY PRESS

OXFORD

UNIVERSITY PRESS

Great Clarendon Street, Oxford OX2 6DP

Oxford University Press is a department of the University of Oxford.
It furthers the University's objective of excellence in research, scholarship,
and education by publishing worldwide in

Oxford New York

Auckland Cape Town Dar es Salaam Hong Kong Karachi
Kuala Lumpur Madrid Melbourne Mexico City Nairobi
New Delhi Shanghai Taipei Toronto

With offices in

Argentina Austria Brazil Chile Czech Republic France Greece
Guatemala Hungary Italy Japan Poland Portugal Singapore
South Korea Switzerland Thailand Turkey Ukraine Vietnam

Oxford is a registered trade mark of Oxford University Press
in the UK and in certain other countries

Published in the United States
by Oxford University Press Inc., New York

© Oxford University Press, 2011

British Library Cataloging in Publication Data

Data available

Library of Congress Cataloging in Publication Data

Data available

Typeset in Minion by Glyph International, Bangalore, India
Printed in Great Britain
on acid-free paper by
CPI Antony Rowe, Chippenham, Wiltshire

ISBN 978–0–19–954479–0

10 9 8 7 6 5 4 3 2 1

Contents

The authors

Martin Plant was the main author of this book and of its sister publication, *Binge Britain*. Sadly, Martin died in early 2010 shortly after completing this manuscript. He was Professor of Addiction Studies in the Alcohol and Health Research Unit at the University of the West of England, Bristol, UK. Prior to that he was Professor in the Alcohol Research Group, later the Alcohol and Health Research Group, at the University of Edinburgh before setting up an independent charity, the Alcohol and Health Research Trust. His publication quality and rate was impressive, including hundreds of articles in peer-reviewed journals as well as a number of books including *Drugtakers in an English Town* (1975), *Drugs in Perspective* (1981, 1987), *Risktakers: Alcohol, Drugs, Sex and Youth* (1992), *Alcohol: Minimising the Harm* (1997), *The Alcohol Report* (2000), and *Binge Britain: Alcohol & the National Response* (2006). He was co-editor of *Alcohol Problems in Employment* (1981), *Economics and Alcohol* (1983), *Alcohol-Related Problems in High Risk Groups: Epidemiological Perspectives* (1981), and *AIDS, Drugs and Prostitution: Studies from Four Continents* (1993), as well as a four-volume anthology entitled *Addiction: Major Themes in Health and Welfare* (2007). He was Director of the UK part of the European School Survey Project on Alcohol & other Drugs (ESPAD). His special interests included the epidemiology of alcohol and other drugs and the effectiveness of and barriers to the implementation of policy options.

Roy Robertson is Honorary Clinical Reader in the Division of Community Health Sciences at the University of Edinburgh. He has worked as a full-time National Health Service general practitioner for many years in a deprived area of Edinburgh. He has directed the long-running Edinburgh Drug Addiction Study and is an acknowledged authority on illicit drugs and HIV/AIDS. He has served on the Advisory Council on the Misuse of Drugs as well as committees of the Department of Health, the Home Office, and the Scottish Executive. He was Chairman of the Shipman Committee. Roy currently holds a grant from the Chief Scientist Office to research the long-term effects of injecting-drug use. He has been a trainer in General Practice and an advisor to various parliamentary, criminal justice, media, and educational groups on topics relating to drug misuse, hepatitis C, and HIV/AIDS. His publications include the book *Heroin, AIDS and Society*. Roy Robertson is Apothecary to the Royal Household at the Palace of Holyrood in Edinburgh.

Moira Plant is Professor of Alcohol Studies at the University of the West of England, Bristol. She is also director of the Alcohol and Health Research Unit. Her publications include the books *Women, Drinking and Pregnancy* and *Women and Alcohol: Contemporary and Historical Perspectives* as well as numerous articles in peer reviewed journals. With her husband Martin she co-authored a number of books including *Risk-takers: Alcohol, Drugs, Sex and Youth,* and *Binge Britain: Alcohol and the National Response* winner of "highly commended" (silver) Mental Health Book Award from the British Medical Association. She is Director of the UK and Isle of Man components of Gender, Alcohol and Culture: an International Study (GENACIS). Her main research interests include women and alcohol and alcohol-related foetal harm.

Patrick Miller is Visiting Senior Research Fellow in the Alcohol and Health Research Unit in the University of the West of England, Bristol, UK. He has worked for many years on surveys of substance use in both adults and teenagers. He plays a leading role in analysing and documenting findings from the UK part of the European School Survey Project on Alcohol and other Drugs (ESPAD). Patrick was Chairman of the ESPAD working group on attitudes. He is also a key member of the research team working on Gender, Alcohol and Culture: an International Study (GENACIS) for the UK and the Isle of Man. He has also been involved in studies of schizophrenia and, in particular, in work on life events and depression.

This book is suffused with Martin's enthusiasm and determination to educate and inform a wide public about the hazards, risks, and dangers of drug use as well as the positive and less discussed aspects of drug use. It is also a vintage assessment of the complex social, medical, and political dynamic that sustains drug use and addiction problems in the UK and contains an extraordinary accumulation of wisdom and intelligent observation gathered over several decades at the front line of drug and alcohol research and policy making. For those of us who knew him well he was a fearless observer, and sometimes critic, of drug and alcohol policy. His balanced approach to these complex issues in the international alcohol and drug arena will be greatly missed.

Acknowledgements

Many people have helped in the production of this book. Thanks go to several people for their work, advice, information, and support. These include Professor Bruce Alexander, Mrs Barbara Andersson, Mr Steven Longmire, Dr Philippe Arvers, Professor Christopher Dunn, Dr Elizabeth Fuller, Professor Henk Garretsen, Professor Graeme Hawthorne, Mr Björn Hibell, Mr Barry McCrory, Professor David Nutt, Ms Emma Plant, Professor Christiane Poulain, Dr Peter Rice, and Mr Mike Trace. The production of this book has been generously supported by the University of the West of England, Bristol. Ms Jane Wathen, Mrs Jan Green, and Ms Liza Mccarron are thanked for aiding the production or reproduction of a number of illustrations, figures, and graphs. Some of the material in Chapter 8 has been reproduced or adapted from an unpublished report on cannabis reclassification. This was originally written for the Joseph Rowntree Foundation. In addition, the Joseph Rowntree Foundation kindly supported the analysis presented in Chapter 2 on the subject of the relationship between first drink and teenage substance use. Roger Penwill is thanked for his cartoons. Drugscope, the General Register Office for Scotland, the NHS Information Centre, and the Office for National Statistics are thanked for information. The Health Development Policy Branch, Investing for Health Unit, Population Health Directorate, Department of Health, Social Services and Public Safety, Belfast, the Office of Public Sector Information, and the TSO are thanked for permission to reproduce Crown Copyright information. The Association of Public Health Observatories (APHO) is also thanked for permission to reproduce some statistical information. The authors' past research has been supported by many agencies. These include the University of the West of England, Bristol, charities, research councils, the alcoholic beverage industry, government departments, health care trusts, local authorities, the police, universities, the European Union, and the World Health Organization. The views expressed in this book are those of the authors. They do not necessarily represent any of the people acknowledged here or the agencies that have ever funded their work.

Introduction

Drug Nation is intended for a wide and general readership. It has been written in non-technical terms. It is hoped that this book will provide an accessible and lucid introduction to some of the main health and social issues related to 'illicit drugs' and their use in the UK. These themes will include a description of drugs such as amphetamines, cannabis, cocaine, ecstasy (MDMA), heroin, and LSD and the law related to such substances. The book offers a discussion of the types of positive and negative effects associated with drug use. A number of very detailed and weighty documents have been produced about drugs in the UK in recent years. Some of these are excellent, or are at least extremely thoughtful and thought-provoking.

    Drug Nation does not set out to review all of these in minute detail because they are worth reading in their complete and original forms. Even so, *Drug Nation* does aim to provide a guide to evidence (including the findings of European School Survey Project on Alcohol and other Drugs (ESPAD), a major new UK survey of teenagers) concerning patterns of drug use and drug-related problems in the UK as well as to indicate the nature of some of the recent drug debates. Drug use is considered in relation to the consequences of use and the conflicting tensions between policies intended to help those with drug problems and to curb or eradicate drug use. Illicit drug use is the subject of a fierce, acrimonious, intolerant, and highly polarized debate. This relates to both the morality and acceptability of drug use as well as the objectives of policy and the options to attain its goals. This debate has frequently been highly irrational and dishonest. It overshadows national and international policies on all aspects of drug use. *Drug Nation* also presents a highly critical review of issues related to the massive impact of drugs on the criminal justice system. A review is also presented of current evidence related to the effectiveness of drug treatment and drug control policies. The latter include largely ineffective drug education and 'shock horror' media campaigning and excessive reliance upon law enforcement and the criminal justice system. It will be argued that UK drug policy is strongly driven by misconceptions, prejudice, panic, and myth. Priorities for a more effective and balanced, evidence-led, approach to illicit drugs are suggested.

Chapter 1

Drugs in Britain: the history

The intentional use of mind-altering substances by humans has a very long history:

> to the conventional view, humans have shared a co-evolutionary relationship with psychotropic plant substances that is millions of years old. We argue that this 'deep time' relationship is self-evident both in the extant chemical–ecological adaptations that have evolved in mammals to metabolize psychotropic plant substances and in the structure of plant defensive chemicals that have evolved to mimic the structure, and interfere with the function, of mammalian neurotransmitters. Given this evidence, we question how emotional mechanisms easily triggered by plant toxins can have evolved. Our argument is also supported with archeological and historical evidence of substance use in antiquity suggesting that, for people in the past, psychotropic plant substances were as much a mundane everyday item as they are for many people today. Our second, and more speculative, objective is to suggest provisional hypotheses of human substance-using phenomena that can incorporate the evolutionary implications of a deep time relationship between psychotropic substances and people.
>
> (Sullivan and Hagen 2002, p.389)

Hallucinogenic drugs are among the oldest drugs used by human beings. These drugs are available naturally in mushrooms, cacti, poppies, and other plants.

Humans have been using psychoactive (mind-altering) drugs since ancient times. The earliest cultural evidence of cannabis (marihuana/marijuana) use originates from the Neolithic era in China, over 6000 years ago. There is also evidence of other ancient drug use during the Neolithic period. Opium appears to have been used in ancient Babylon both to relieve pain and to bring on sleep. During more recent times opium and its derivatives (such as laudanum) have been widely used in medicine. Before the introduction of anaesthesia during the nineteenth century, a mixture of opium and alcohol was extensively used to stupefy surgical patients and to shield them from the pain of operations. Opium was also widely used recreationally throughout much of Britain. In fact, social attitudes to psychoactive drugs have often, if not usually, been ambivalent. Substances such as opium and cannabis have been used recreationally in Britain for centuries and a significant percentage of the population was thought to be dependent on laudanum at the end of the nineteenth century. This chapter will provide a historical insight into the important role of such substances in British society. It will consider the ambivalent, often highly moralizing, social response to a growing phenomenon. This review will chart the rise of illicit drug use from its apparent origins as an unusual practice to become widespread and normalized throughout much of the UK.

> It begins when 'drug' becomes 'dope.' In the nineteenth century, it was understood that certain middle class women and professional men had the 'drug habit.' These were seen as individual burdens, though: the unfortunate by-products of medical treatment, or unwise attempts to cope with the demands of brain-work. Private weaknesses like these did not lead to serious restrictions on the availability of opiates or cocaine, let alone the criminalisation of their non-medical use. Once the 'dope fiend' was identified as a species, however, drugs came to be regarded as properly a police matter. The outlawing of drugs was the consequence, not of their pharmacology, but of their association with social groups perceived as potentially dangerous.
>
> (Plant and Plant 1992, p.2)

Roman Britain and before

Human-like beings may have intermittently been present in parts of what is now Britain (glaciations permitting) for 700 000 years. 'Boxgrove Man' (*Homo heidelbergensis*), probably an ancestor of both Neanderthals and our own species, lived in the region of the modern town of Chichester 500 000 years ago (Stringer 2006). These beings were tool-using hunters. Their teeth suggest that they were adapted to eat food such as fruit as well as meat (Stringer and Andrews 2005). If this is so, then it is possible that these early Britons, like some other mammals, may have eaten some forms of psychoactive plants, such as fungi, berries, or fermented fruit. They may have experienced and enjoyed their effects. Nevertheless, the subject of animals such as elephants allegedly deliberately seeking intoxication has certainly been sensationalized and exaggerated (Morris et al. 2006). McKenna (1992) advanced what has been called the 'stoned ape' theory. This speculated (to the likely horror of creationists) that the evolution of the modern human consciousness may have been facilitated by the consumption of drugs such as psilocybin contained in wild fungi. A 60 000-year-old Neanderthal burial site in Northern Iraq has been found to contain remnants of ephedra, a herbal stimulant. It is unknown whether the presence of this herb signified a burial ritual, the religious significance of the herb, or even recreational drug use. It has, however, been speculated that the plants found at this and similar sites were used for their remedial properties (Lietava 1992, Norton 2005, New Scientist 2006). Neanderthals are no longer with us. What is not in doubt is that modern humans have used mind-altering drugs for thousands of years:

> Hunter gather cultures—without doubt the oldest ones on the planet—have in common an open and endless plurality of gods. We know that in a great majority of those societies, subjects learn and reaffirm their cultural identity through experience with psychoactive drugs. Such traditions constitute, therefore, a very basic chapter, often forgotten until recently, of what would be called revealed truth by later religions, more suited to sedentary cultures…. The first host or holy sacraments were psychoactive substances such as peyote, wine, or certain fungi.
>
> (Escohatado 1999, p.2)

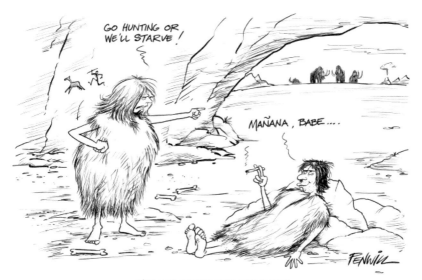

THE END OF THE NEANDERTHALS

Credit: Roger Penwill.

The chronology of at least some forms of drug use has been evident since the beginnings of agriculture approximately 10 000 years ago:

> Some evidence that the first crops included psychoactive plants such as mandrake, tobacco, coffee and cannabis…
> 7,000 BC—Betel seeds chewed for their stimulant effects, found in archaeological sites in Asia…
> 6,000 BC—Native South Americans begin cultivating and using tobacco…
> 4,200 BC—Opium poppy seed pods found in a burial site at Albuñol near Granada, Spain…

3,500 BC—Bronze Age vessels show evidence of wine consumption in eastern Mediterranean…

3,000 BC—Cannabis cultivation in China and Asia…

2,000 BC—Coca residues found in hair of Andean mummies…

1,000 BC—Central Americans erect temples to mushroom gods…

800 BC—Distillation of spirits in India.

430 BC—Greek historian Heroditus records recreational cannabis smoking among the Scythian people of the Black Sea.

(New Scientist 2006)

The cultivation of opium poppies was recorded 5000 years ago on Sumerian tablets. Evidence of hemp use dates from a similar period. Escohatado notes that the use of drug-bearing plants such as 'henbane, nightshade, datura and mandrake' dates back to ancient times and that the use of hallucinogenic plants was evident thousands of years ago in the Americas:

> Pure stimulants, based on drugs such as caffeine and cocaine, also trace their history to ancient times. The coca bush originated in the Andes, and since the third century B.C. there have been sculptures of faces enlarged by chewing coca leaves. Guarná and mate, both of which contain caffeine, are also American, as is cacao, which contains theobromine, a similar substance. Equivalent effects are obtained in India and Indonesia thanks to betel, a drug little known in the West, which is chewed by a tenth of the world's population today. In China, tea, which contains caffeine and tannin, has been used for four or five millennia, as well as ephedra, a much more concentrated stimulant. From Africa come the cola nut, a common caffeine stimulant on the western coast, and khat, a bush consumed in Yemen, Somalia and Ethiopia.

(Escohatado 1999, p 9)

Researchers have found equipment (in the form of ceramic bowls) that was apparently used to prepare a hallucinogenic drug (probably cohoba) for sniffing on the Caribbean island of Carriacou dating back as far as 1000–400 BC (Fitzpatrick et al. 2009).

An earthenware pot discovered at Skara Brae in the Orkneys seems to have been used for drinking beer or other type of alcoholic beverage. The remains at this site are believed to be up to 5000 years old. In addition, a number of Bronze Age cups and chalices, apparently for alcohol, have been found in Britain that originate from 2200–1500 BC. The British love/hate relationship with alcohol has been noted for hundreds of years. Commentators have described, often in scathing terms, the British propensity to drink to excess. It has been noted that this, while by no means unique, is still striking by international standards. Heavy drinking has long been associated with poverty, ill health, and a variety of social problems (Musto 1997, Plant and Plant 2006). Both the ancient Greeks and the Romans (as well as their contemporaries in other societies) were reportedly avid users of recreational drugs, often mixing these with wine (Hillman 2008). They also inhaled drugs:

> Greeks and Romans intentionally exposed themselves to the vapors of burning plants during the practice of "fumigation," a process whereby the drug user breathed in the fumes of various substances, anything from ordinary incense to potent herbs. This was a commonplace activity in recreational, religious and medical settings.
>
> (Hillman 2008, p.59)

It is evident that psychoactive drug use was both well known and widely practised in the classical world. Such substances were known to range from mild and low risk to powerful and potentially dangerous. Hillman has noted that many historical and mythical classical writings cite some drugs that cannot be identified with any certainty. They refer to effects such as pain reduction, disinhibition, conviviality, remorse, disorientation, suicide, insanity, and 'raving' as well as 'euphoria, giddiness and hallucinations'.

> Drugs may have been a potent coping mechanism for tired generals, and eastern potentates, but the pharmaceutical promise of euphoria had its limits in antiquity—just as it does today. That is, our texts show that the Classical world was well aware of the phenomenon known as tolerance. Theophrastus warned his readers of this easily observable fact: "The virtues (powers) of all drugs become weaker to those who are accustomed to them, and in some cases become entirely ineffective."
>
> (Hillman 2008, p.63)

Interestingly, Hillman (whose book *The Chemical Muse* is fascinating, not least for its shocking insight into a recent example of deplorable academic politics and narrow-mindedness) reports that classical writing about drugs sometimes criticized untrustworthy suppliers, but appeared to lack pejorative terms for the users themselves.

The Romans used henbane, wormwood, cannabis, and opium both medicinally and recreationally. They almost certainly used these while occupying large areas of Britain. Moreover, drugs from indigenous plants (such as 'magic mushrooms') have probably been used in this country for thousands of years, regardless of the arrival and departure of Roman armies.

The Middle Ages

Martin (2008) notes that:

> Cannabis was probably being used as a recreational drug when Shakespeare was writing, and he may have made a cryptic reference to it in his work.
>
> (Martin 2008, p.53)

This alludes to a reference to 'a noted weed' and 'compounds strange' in Sonnet 76. Martin also cites other evidence of more cannabis use. This took the form of the: 'possible chemical residues of cannabis in the remnants of seventeenth-century clay pipes that were recovered from the site of Shakespeare's house in Stratford upon Avon'. Opium was available in Britain during Shakespeare's time. It has also, surprisingly, been suggested that 'cocaine' (or presumably coca) was also in evidence, long before it became widely known in Europe. (The cocaine alkaloid was first isolated in 1855.)

The eighteenth and nineteenth centuries

The 'gin craze' of the eighteenth century is one of the most notorious periods in the British history of using mind-altering drugs. For decades heavy gin consumption was recognized as causing major health and social problems, especially among the urban poor. Governments responded to this situation by liberalizing the sale of beer and by badly enforced attempts at taxing gin. In the end, the enforcement of more reasonable taxes appeared to contribute to the reduction of this problem (Musto 1997, Warner 2003).

In Scotland in the nineteenth century large quantities of whisky were consumed. In the 1830s it was estimated that two and a half gallons of legally distilled spirit were consumed per head of population, and quantities of illicit whisky were also drunk (Smout and Wood 1991, p.147).

The Romantic Poets (Byron, Keats, Shelley, Coleridge, and Wordsworth) were all as notorious for their allegedly dissolute, drug-using lifestyles as any modern rock stars. Their drugs of preference were laudanum (an opium-based painkiller) and gin (Andronik 2007). Laudanum was also widely used by working-class people, since it was cheaper than gin. The joys (and problems) associated with opium were vividly described by De Quincey in a series of articles in the *London Magazine* in 1821. This narrative is best known as *Confessions of an Opium Eater* (see De Quincey 1995). Samuel Taylor Coleridge, one of the Lakes Poets and a friend of De Quincey, was dependent upon opium. During some stages of his life he claimed that this aided his writing, while at other times he denigrated the harm that its use had inflicted upon him. His opium scales are on display in William Wordsworth's cottage in Grasmere (Lefebure 1974).

Opium was uncontrolled, available, and widely used as both a medicine and an intoxicant throughout Britain during the eighteenth and nineteenth centuries. Poppy cultivation was popular. Successful growers (some of whom were medical practitioners) even won prizes at horticultural shows. The use of opium and poppy tea was famously commonplace in the fenland area of

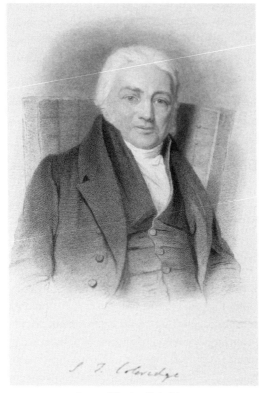

Samuel Taylor Coleridge
Credit: AP/Press Association Images.

East Anglia during the nineteenth century. The British Medical Association estimated that half of Britain's considerable opium imports were consumed in this area, together with domestically grown opium:

> The subsequent social changes which led to greater integration of the area into the rest of the country may have contributed to a decline in this practice. In recent years poppy tea drinking has been revived within the illicit drug using community and a survey using a self-report questionnaire was carried out among patients attending the Cambridge Drug Dependency Unit. Forty-three patients admitted to drinking poppy tea, usually during the summer months and on an intermittent basis.
>
> (London et al. 2006, p.1345)

Opium use has been ably reviewed by Berridge (1999). She notes that opium was widely used in Western medicine by the sixteenth century.

> In England the drug had early been used, chiefly for its narcotic properties.... The drug's soporific and narcotic qualities reappear in Chaucer's Canterbury Tales and

in Shakespeare, in particular in the famous passage from Othello: "Not poppy, nor mandragore, Nor all the drowsy syrups of the world, Shall ever medicine thee to that sweet sleep Which thou ow'dst yesterday."

(Berridge 1999, p. xxiii)

Berridge notes that at the beginning of the nineteenth century opium was viewed as a useful medicine. It was on sale legally and was widely available. She also reports that regular users, or 'opium eaters', were:

acceptable in their communities and rarely the subject of medical attention at the beginning of the century; at its end they were classified as 'sick,' diseased or deviant in some way and fit subjects for professional treatment.

(Berridge 1999, p.xxix)

This total redefinition was probably attributable to the problems that ensued from uncontrolled availability and widespread use. Moreover, doctors and pharmacists, as noted by Berridge, were increasingly defining opium use as a medical phenomenon. Opium was extensively used as a medicine, to treat a wide variety of ailments such as mental illness, diabetes, malaria, and cholera. Some medicines used mixtures of opium and alcohol. There is no doubt that many people also used opium recreationally. As was the case with gin drinking, the problem appears to have been largely defined in relation to opium used by working-class people. Berridge also reported that fears of working-class opium use were compounded by alarm at the use of this drug by Chinese people in dockside areas. The availability of opium was restricted by the Pharmacy Act of 1868:

The restrictions of the 1868 Act—the 'professionalization' of the sale of patent medicines and the curbs on prescription—were part of the establishment of a professional elite. Once the 'stimulant' scare was over, working-class drug use was largely ignored. Instead ... doctors concentrated on the question of hypodermic morphine, where a small number of injecting addicts were magnified by the medical perspective on the drug into the dimensions of a pressing problem.

(Berridge 1999, p xxxi)

The history of drugs is well supplied with odd characters. One of these was the notorious (and vaguely sinister, or maybe just a bit sad) Aliester Crowley, author of the novel *Diary of a Drug Fiend* (1922). Crowley, mountaineer, occultist, and writer, was notorious for a wide-ranging drug experimentation (laudanum, opium, hashish, cocaine, mescalin, and heroin) that was in many ways ahead of its time.

The modern Royal Navy features its drug interdiction (interception) activities as part of its recruitment publicity. This has not always been so. The Scottish trading company Jardine Matheson's early profits were based on the sale of Indian opium in China. The ruling Qing Dynasty attempted to ban this trade which actively promoted drug dependence in China. In response to this threat to its profits, the company appealed to the British Government to force China to permit opium trading. The Chinese resisted, but were defeated militarily after the two inglorious Opium Wars (1839–1842 and 1856–1860). These conflicts ended with China being forced into signing the so-called Unequal Treaties. These, among other things, ceded Hong Kong to Britain. The Chinese opium trade was paralleled by enormous British profiteering from the cannabis trade in India. Cannabis was used in Britain for medicinal purposes (such as emotional problems, headaches, and heavy menstrual bleeding). Even so, it appears not to have been widely taken as a recreational drug in this country during the nineteenth century (Mills 2003). It is ironic that the Royal Navy, now a very active enforcer of drug control, once acted to serve the interests of opium traders.

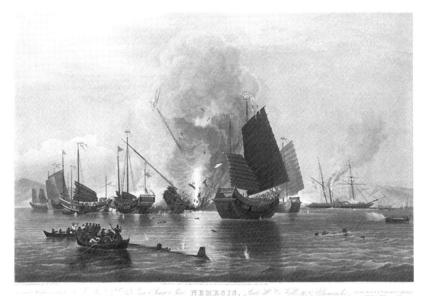

HMS Nemesis destroying Chinese war junks, First Opium War, 1841
Credit: Edward Duncan 1843.

Arguably, the forerunner of a series of acts of Parliament related to attempting to control the production, distribution, or sale of 'dangerous drugs' in the UK was the Poisons Act (1858). This legislation, a follow-up to the more limited Arsenic Act of 1851, restricted and controlled the supply of poisonous substances.

This legislation was mainly introduced to prevent poisons from being obtained by potential murderers. This legislation formed the basis of what over time developed into the UK's contemporary drug-control laws. The latter are elaborated upon in Chapter 5.

The twentieth century

By the beginning of the twentieth century certain types of drug use had already been defined as constituting 'problems'. During the First World War, London's Commissioner of Police reported that cocaine was being sold, allegedly by prostitutes and military personnel. Legislation to curb this practice was introduced in the form of the Defence of the Realm Act (1916). These measures were strengthened in 1917 and yet again by the Dangerous Drugs Act (1920). These measures broadened legislation to include all substances covered by the First International Opium Convention of 1912.

Berridge has argued as follows:

> The international control system which did so much to form domestic policies in the 1920s began life simply as an attempt to control opiate use and trade in the Far East, as part also of American trade expansion in that area.

(Berridge 1999, p.xxxii)

After the Second World War it was evident that some returning military personnel had adopted cannabis smoking while abroad. There was also a rise in the use of heroin. The existing small and stable group of people who received opiate drugs on prescription was augmented by young people who used heroin recreationally. An American-style 'drug scene' was beginning to develop. In 1958, the Brain Committee was convened to consider the situation. This body produced a remarkably reassuring report (Interdepartmental Committee on Drug Addiction 1961). Shortly after the release of this document Home Office figures revealed a big rise in recorded heroin dependence. The situation was changing. Cannabis use was spreading and drugs were beginning to rise on the nation's agenda. The Brain Committee was reconvened and produced a second report (Interdepartmental Committee on Drug Addiction 1965). This concluded that there had been an alarming increase in 'drug misuse' since 1961. Popular alarm about the use of illicit drugs was compounded by concern at another new phenomenon: the rise of youth culture and the associated emergence of 'the teenager'. During the 1950s considerable publicity was devoted to the activities of gangs of 'Teddy boys', at least some of whom were reputed to be heavy recreational users of amphetamines. The Teddy boys, distinguished by their 'Edwardian' manner of dress and quiff or pompadour hairstyles, combined an enthusiasm for US-style rock and roll music and drug use.

They were simply the first wave of what has been a succession of youthful fads, often combining music, styles of dress, and taste in drugs. Teddy boys were succeeded by Mods and Rockers, Hippies, Punks, and Goths. The high point of youth culture and the associated drug scene is regarded by many people (including at least one of the authors) as the 1960s and 1970s. The conflicts between gangs of Mods and Rockers during the 1960s (often at seaside towns such as Clacton) was reported extensively and often in an exaggerated and sensational manner. The social scientist Stanley Cohen (1972) used the term 'moral panic' to describe the lurid manner in which some of the media reported the conflict between Mods and Rockers. This term has periodically been used in relation to other drug-related phenomena as well as other forms of behaviour. Such panics are considered further in Chapter 8. It is worth noting that there is some factual basis for concern in relation to many, if not most, moral panics. Only a minority are conjured out of thin air. An exaggerated social response does not mean that nothing is really happening. The 1960s set the scene for the growth and establishment of recreational drug use occurring in the context of the distinctive leisure and lifestyles of teenagers and young adults. This phenomenon arose partly in imitation of developments (rock and roll and Hippies) evident in the USA, but assumed home-grown characteristics and styles (e.g. Mods, Skinheads, and Punks) which influenced not only the youth of North America, but those in many other countries.

> If you can remember the sixties, you probably weren't there.

Do you remember or have you heard about the 'summer of love?' This refers to 1967 when people flocked to the Haight-Ashbury neighbourhood of San Franciso for a hedonistic celebration of drugs combined with sexual and political freedom. This highlighted the link between recreational drug use with Hippy 'counterculture'. A vast amount has been written about the rise and rise of youth culture (e.g. Abrams 1959, Roberts 1983, Halsey 1986, Thornton 1996).

It is not proposed to reiterate this here. Even so, it should be emphasized that illicit drug use cannot be understood without an awareness of the driving force of increasingly globalized styles of consumption and leisure, particularly among young people (Alexander 2008).

It has been evident that the use of cannabis in particular has been so widespread for so long that it has become 'normalized' (Measham et al. 1994, Parker et al. 1998, Parker 2005). While it is true that illicit drugs have been and are used by many people in the UK, their use is still controversial. This is indicated periodically when politicians or other prominent people are asked whether or not they have ever used cannabis or other drugs. Responses to this question include no comment, denial, admission, or statements to the effect that they had used but did not inhale or did not enjoy the effects:

> Conservative leader David Cameron has refused to deny claims in a biography that he smoked cannabis while he was a pupil at Eton College 25 years ago.
>
> (BBC News Online, 11 February, 2007a)

> A string of Cabinet ministers have owned up to smoking cannabis after Home Secretary Jacqui Smith said she had used the drug at Oxford in the 1980s. Chancellor Alistair Darling and Transport Secretary Ruth Kelly are among those to admit using the drug when they were younger. Prime Minister Gordon Brown was among those to say they had never used it.
>
> (BBC News Online, 20 July, 2007c)

Chapter 2

Drugs in perspective

In a book about the nature and impact of drug taking it is important to spend some time discussing the range and nature of the drugs involved. This chapter provides what is hoped to be an accessible description of drug dependence or 'addiction' and the chemical and pharmacological effects of the main illicit substances that are used recreationally the UK. These substances include amphetamines, cannabis (including 'skunk'), cocaine, crack, ecstasy (MDMA), LSD, heroin, opium, and morphine.

Descriptive problems start at the very beginning, however. The word 'drug' means different things to different people and can refer to any active molecule having an effect on the individual who is consuming it. It conjures up numerous visions ranging from plant and herbal substances to medicinal medications and illicit addictive compounds, the range of which seems to increase all the time. A drug is variously seen as life-saving therapy, a trial and experimental intervention, a personal indulgence, or a substance associated with compulsive and uncontrolled dependence or, in some contexts, a poison. Foodstuffs may be classified as a drug and active compounds, known as drugs, may be synthetic or naturally occurring. New and effective pharmaceutical drugs developed over the last three or four decades by industry are, to some extent, responsible for the increase in years of life expectancy in many countries. The investment and development in the drug-producing pharmaceutical industry is seen by most people as important and is, of course, a massive part of the economy of many Western countries. Conversely pharmaceuticals can be seen at times as a threat to a more 'natural' lifestyle. The need for drugs of all sorts is usually recognized by all of us even if the apparent contradictions are complex. It is perhaps unfortunate that there are so many meanings and interpretations contained in the word 'drug'.

Drugs are, therefore, everywhere in modern life. They are part of our diet, important for normal metabolism, and responsible for increasing longevity. However, they can be harmful and that is the subject of this chapter. Harm can be caused by the accidental or misguided use of drugs. Frequent mistakes are attributed to doctors and nurses administering inappropriate or wrong strengths of medicinal drugs and allergies and idiosyncratic reactions account for more damage. The use of self-administered drugs which are harmful is increasing and covers many categories of drugs and many different circumstances. The range of possible drugs with potentially harmful effects is large and the variety of circumstances in which they are taken seems unlimited. The understanding of the most commonly used drugs or compounds is, however, central to management of drug-related problems and any attempt to regulate adverse effects associated with drug use.

Modern pharmacology promises much but has also introduced a complex range of substances which can be used for harm as well as for good. Any compound with a psychoactive effect is likely to be taken for recreational purposes at times and this sometimes seems like an inevitable side effect in the development of any medicine. The pharmaceutical industry and the regulatory authorities are exquisitely aware of the dangers posed when medications are used outside their recommended dose or setting. Effective compounds such as selective serotonin re-uptake inhibitors (SSRIs) are a good example of drugs which have been a significant advance in therapy for depression but also have an abuse potential. Examples of this group are fluoxetine (Prozac), paroxetine, and citalopram, drugs which can also induce a sense of well-being in individuals without any identifiable illness. This raises the question of the use of compounds such as these to enhance moods and, arguably, to improve life for those taking the drug without harmful effect. The prospect of a new generation of life-enhancing drugs with no detrimental effect raises moral, ethical, and philosophical questions for individuals, policy makers, and legislators. Boundaries have arisen in the public consciousness between damaging drugs, drugs which have only a small perceived risk, and those which may have few harmful effects but are restricted and which, to others, represent harm in a wider sense of that consequent on lifestyles that are antisocial or limiting in other ways. Debates over widespread use, verging on 'normal behaviour', in some sectors of society have been active over drugs such as ecstasy, cannabis and cocaine. It is not hard to observe the inconsistency between the 'legal' use of a bewildering array of alcohol-related products which are associated with considerable morbidity and mortality and the so-called recreational drugs which are illegal but which, at times, seem to cause less harm. The debate over the appropriate use of legislation and control over drug availability will, continue with powerful arguments to support all views but in an arena where politicians fear to tread and where they find little opportunity for support from the electorate. This debate is considered in detail later in this book. The firm line and strong legislation and control approach has served political parties well over many years. A united policy on control of drug supply and use has been seen as important by the international community and the need for consensus between nations is unlikely to allow a mellowing in the legal constraints. United Nations charters governing these controls are important backgrounds to domestic laws (United Nations 1961, 1971, 1988).

Some important terms

Terminology is widely used in the popular press and media and most people have an understanding of the commonly used terms 'addiction', 'dependence', 'withdrawal', 'tolerance', 'recovery' and 'abstinence'. Because they are used frequently and are in everyday speech, interpretation is at times confused and the same term can mean slightly different things to different people. The word 'depression', for example, has a variety of meanings to different people ranging from sadness and upset over a trivial issue to a serious and even life-threatening illness associated with delusional thoughts and withdrawal from normal life, requiring invasive hospital treatment. Similarly, addiction can be viewed as common and trivial or as life-threatening and serious. People will often say that they are addicted to chocolate, coffee, or behaviours such as gambling, Internet use, sex, exercise, or sport (Plant and Plant 2008).

Many of the features of damaging addiction are shared by these situations. For most of us, however, the word 'addiction' is associated with damaging and at times illegal behaviour. Addiction is also commonly referred to as dependence or dependent drug use and has several formal definitions. Most include the features of compulsive use over a period of time which is often associated with withdrawal on cessation and is characterized by increasing tolerance to the drug in question. However, addiction or dependence is more complicated than a simple physical state and is usually attended by a psychological dependence equally as damaging as the physical state of dependence. In many cases psychological dependence is the dominant feature and it is most often the cause of relapse into drug taking after a period of abstinence. Most people recognize the psychological state of dependence and the alterations it can cause in personality and behaviour. Indeed it is now increasingly thought that a permanent altered brain function may be present in those chronically dependent patients which precludes easy reversal to a drug-free lifestyle. Withdrawal symptoms are, again, widely recognized and experiences of withdrawal from the effect of alcohol are familiar to most people. Withdrawal from most drugs have different effects and depend to a certain extent on the length of time the drug has been used, the quantity taken and the psychological state of the individual. Withdrawal from strong opiates are very rare in the case of an individual who is otherwise inexperienced with the drug and requires it for a short period for pain relief under medical supervision. Tolerance is absent, psychological dependence is not a problem, and once the pain is relieved there is no further requirement for the drug. Withdrawal in the chronically dependent person with a high capacity and tolerance and a profound psychological dependence are quite different and can be dramatic and distressing. Interesting examples of people previously dependent on opiates and other drugs experiencing marked withdrawal symptoms when being in a situation associated with drug taking but without taking any drug show the power of psychological dependence. The brain retains a memory of the dependent state strong enough to trigger the symptoms of rapid heartbeat, sweating, and even the pleasurable features of the drug.

Tolerance is an important feature of dependence on drugs. After repeated use of a drug the body develops a familiarity to the effects on the receptors and larger doses are required to achieve similar effects. This effect is different for different drugs and seemingly in different individuals and can develop at different rates depending upon quantity or frequency of use, the type of drug, and the biochemical makeup of the individual. It is therefore difficult to measure and dangerously difficult to depend upon. Loss of tolerance can happen fairly quickly after abstinence, resulting in dangerous and unexpected overdose when resuming drug taking at the previously tolerated amount. The commonly recognized example of this is the danger of fatal overdose in people released from custody and resuming drug taking at their previous level after an abstinent period.

Abstinence is a term of great contemporary interest not least by policy makers and politicians eager to define recovery and measure improvement. Abstinence may mean the absence of drugs over a short or long period, or, for some, the complete cessation of intake over a long time. Similarly, recovery means, for some, the development of an equilibrium and steady state of improvement. Others would define recovery as complete and long-term abstinence from the drug with the expectation that any future drug taking would not happen. For some experts and observers recovery can be associated with a steady state on some treatment programme and not necessarily by abstinence from all drugs. For example, the opiate drug user who has taken no heroin for months or years but takes the substitute methadone and still smokes cigarettes and sometimes cannabis would be said, by some, to be recovered or in recovery. Others would say any drug use precludes the definition recovery. A useful definition of recovery was recently published by the UK Drug Policy Commission (UKDPC 2008):

> The process of recovery is characterised by voluntarily sustained control over substance use which maximises health and well-being and participation in the rights, roles and responsibilities of society.

(www.ukdpc.org.uk)

The drugs that cause concern

The most widely used recreational drug in Western cultures is, of course, beverage alcohol. This is associated with many more deaths than all other psychoactive drugs with the exception of tobacco. A quote from a recent influential report sums up the damage done.

> Doctors are often unaware of the contribution of alcohol to the cause of death and, even when they are, they may be unwilling to attach the stigma of alcohol to the deceased when signing death certificates. Within these constraints, estimates of the number of alcohol-related deaths per year in Britain have varied from 5000 to 40 000.

(Royal College of Physicians 2001a)

Since that report concerns have increased, especially in relation to young people drinking heavily. Estimates of liver damage in the future have increased dramatically (Plant and Plant 2006, British Medical Association 2008, NHS Confederation 2010). The scale of adverse drug effects is considered further in Chapter 4.

Alcohol, despite the portrayal as otherwise in popular culture, is a central nervous system depressant and is, in a dose-related effect, a sedative. It has a disinhibiting effect and induces a feeling of well-being in many but in some people the opposite. It has a well-known social effect and has attributed to it, although with a contradictory evidence base, a positive effect on health for middle-aged and older people. In the short term it has many adverse features including gastrointestinal upset (nausea and diarrhoea), confusion and irrational behaviour, disinhibition leading to aggressive, violent and antisocial behaviour and poor judgement. In the longer term it is responsible for addiction, organ damage, mental problems, and social damage.

This chapter is not principally about alcohol, but it is important to note that its impact is increasing and that it is often used in combination with illegal drugs with serious consequences. Many of the deaths attributed to illegal drugs are noted to occur in the presence of alcohol. Combined overdosage may at least in a proportion of these cases have led to a death which would not have occurred without alcohol. Also contributory may be the disorganization and disinhibition caused by the coexisting alcohol use and the combined important effect of other drugs and alcohol on respiration and response rates. Alcohol therefore causes collateral damage as well as morbidity related to its own toxicity. Nowhere is this clearer than the disastrous effects of driving when under the influence of alcohol. Many illegal drug users resort to alcohol in a later phase of their lives and display similar dependency characteristics in its use that they did with illegal drugs. In treatment situations and in crisis management addressing the alcohol problem may be as important if not more important than the illegal drug problem. Services are increasingly trying to combine these treatment services.

Tobacco occupies a similar position to alcohol in the aetiology of disease and in the treatment situation. Although the damaging effects of smoking have been known about for more than 50 years it is still one of the most common causes of death due to self administration of a toxin (Doll and Bradford Hill 1954). Clearly a legal drug, tobacco is, paradoxically, responsible for many times the death rate attributable to alcohol and dramatically more than that mortality ascribed to illegal drugs. In most years in the UK there may be 100 000 deaths directly related to tobacco, up to 40 000 caused by alcohol, and 'only' 3000 or so related directly to illegal drugs. Despite these extraordinary statistics policy and practice seem unable to acknowledge the disproportionate allocation of attention given to illegal drugs and the relative success in illegal drug treatment compared to the increasing damage caused by alcohol and tobacco. As well as failure at government level the reckless and uncontrollable encouragement of use of these drugs allowed by the commercial interest of the tobacco and alcohol industries continues to surprise those interested in public health and clinical care. Tobacco is a drug which is highly addictive, and dependency usually develops some time after the onset of use but is persistent and extraordinarily difficult to overcome even in the face of increasing education about its damaging effects and opportunities for help with cessation. The most serious consequence of its long-term use is lung cancer, which develops after many years of use and which clearly has a genetic component in its occurrence. There are some people who, in the well-known observation, can smoke 20 cigarettes or more each day and live to be 80 or older. Unfortunately, or maybe fortunately, it is impossible to know which genetic makeup will protect or predispose an individual to cancer. Lung cancer remains at this time one of the cancers with the poorest prognosis and with the least effective treatments.

Interestingly, research has shown that the risk of lung cancer decreases progressively after cessation (although never returning to the risk for someone who has never smoked). This is true even after many years of smoking. Depressingly, smoking rates in women have increased in recent decades and lung cancer in women may well overtake that in men over the next decade in the UK. On a worldwide scale developing countries have shown a relentless increase in tobacco consumption as the tobacco industry targets new markets as regulations and legal consequences discourage marketing in developed countries. It seems incredible to read that the epidemic of lung cancer, heart disease, and pulmonary obstruction deaths caused by smoking cigarettes through the twentieth century in the Western world will unfold in developing countries over the next few decades. The burden of these diseases will be onerous in China, the East, and Africa as smoking rates increase in these countries.

The remainder of this chapter will be devoted to those other drugs commonly considered to be substances that are potentially harmful and addictive. The list shown in Table 2.1 is not exhaustive and the emphasis on and the importance of individual drugs changes year by year as their popularity, and availability, vary. Whilst the use of drugs is determined by simple factors such as availability and fashion the importance of drugs to the public and

Table 2.1 Examples of drugs in different categories

Category	Examples
Opiates	Diamorphine (heroin)
	Morphine
	Methadone
	Codeine and codeine derivatives such as dihydrocodeine
	Codeine combinations (usually with paracetamol)
	Burprenorphine
	Other opiates such as hydromorphone, dipipanone, pethidine, oxycodone, and tramadol
Stimulants and hallucinogens	Cocaine, amphetamine, and other 'psycho stimulants'
	LSD
	Ecstasy (methylenedioxymethamphetamine, MDMA)
Tranquillizers and sedatives	Benzodiazepines (diazepam, temazepam)
	Major tranquillizers (chlorpromazine, promazine, clozapine, haloperidol, resperidone, sulpiride)
	Barbiturates (largely unavailable in the UK since prescribing restrictions became common in the 1970s)
	Methaqualone (mandrax)
Others (which have individual characteristics as well as effects similar to other categories)	Khat
	Cannabis
	Ketamine
	Solvents
	Phencyclidine
	Mephedrone
	Gammahydroxybutrate (GHB)
	Gammabutyrolactone (GBL)
	Volatile substances of abuse (VSA)

to politicians and policy makers is usually the emergence of side effects or behaviour associated with drugs. For example, the use of ecstasy by youth cultures in Europe and North America in the 1990s attracted changes in legislation and control of a new range of drugs the most extreme of which was classifying ecstasy as a Class A drug under the Misuse of Drugs Act. Similarly cases of fatal overdose of methadone in children of drugs users have created enormous interest by the press and media in increasing controls of this and other prescribed drugs.

As well as the effects of a drug which are based on its pharmacological characteristics there are other important things which contribute to its effect and the potential for harm or damage. The most obvious may be the strength or purity of the substance or simply the quantity consumed. Most harm is essentially dose-related; that is, the damaging effect increases with the amount consumed. This is often associated with the method of production of the drug but is also dependent on the mode of delivery. A drug which is inhaled such as cannabis or cocaine can more rapidly pass into the bloodstream than one which is swallowed and absorbed from the stomach. Most importantly for speed of onset are those drugs taken by intravenous injection. With this mode of entry into the body the effects are sudden and dramatic, occurring within seconds. As well as the effects of the drug, injection also allows for serious side effects such as fatal overdose or, almost equally damaging, the introduction of foreign agents or contaminants, such as bacteria, viruses, and fungi. Drug injection is responsible for most cases of hepatitis C and the majority of cases of HIV and hepatitis B in injecting drug users. Take away injecting and many of the serious consequences of opiate use disappear. Interventions and treatments therefore are targeted at the behaviour around drug use as well as the drug type itself.

Some important drugs

Diamorphine (diacetylmorphine, heroin, smack) is a derivative of opium. It was first synthesized in 1874 and later used widely for pain control until its abuse potential was fully realized. The background to the medical use of diamorphine is important as it has implications for the international control of this drug and its subsequent availability as a treatment option for those addicted.

The UK is one of the very few countries which use diamorphine as an analgesic. Only one or two other countries have this opportunity in their legislative framework. From an international perspective this is important and the historical background is not only complicated but relevant to understanding this unique position. After its discovery by Alder Wright in 1874 it was not marketed until 1898, when marketing was started by Heinrich Dreser, a Germany pharmacologist working with the Bayer pharmaceutical company. Heroin became widely reported as a treatment for cough, bronchitis, tuberculosis, asthma and other conditions. It was said to be free from the side effects associated with morphine, such as nausea and constipation, and was thought to be less likely to cause dependence and to be useful for the treatment of morphine and opium dependence.

However, its position as a drug of addiction in the early twentieth century led to it being withdrawn from pharmacopoeias in many countries including the USA in 1924. Its use, however, continued in the UK where its value as an analgesic and in palliative care was considered unique.

In 1953 the Sixth World Health Assembly in Geneva concluded that 'the abolition of legally produced diacetylmorphine from national pharmacopoeia would facilitate the struggle against its illicit use'. In the following year the United Nations Commission on Narcotic Drugs (CND) voted that all countries should be asked to ban heroin and this was endorsed by the United Nations. Britain abstained from voting in this commission but the Department of Health (after consultation with the Standing Medical Advisory Committee, with representatives from the British Medical Association, the General Medical Council, and the Royal Colleges on the importance of heroin in the practice of medicine) agreed that there were effective substitutes available. The UK therefore was quite happy to conform to the United Nations resolutions and it was planned that no further licence would be issued for manufacturing heroin.

The British Pharmacopoeia Commission also concluded that other drugs should be used for analgesia and with the support of the British Medical Association and the Medical Research Council the entry for diamorphine was excluded from the 1953 edition of the *British Pharmacopoeia*.

In February 1955 the government in the UK announced that heroin would no longer be manufactured for medical purposes in the UK after the end of that year. This would have effectively deleted heroin from the British therapeutic pharmacopoeia, in line with the United Nations resolution urging all governments to limit heroin production and trade to small quantities for scientific purposes only. In response many doctors protested that this move would cause hardship to many patients and violated the principle of clinical freedom. The Minister for Health insisted that consultation with the medical establishment had been carried out but the doctors claimed that the Standing Medical Advisory Committee was not authorized to speak on their behalf. At the annual meeting of the British Medical Association a resolution was passed requesting that the manufacture of heroin should continue and the medical establishment then changed sides and backed the doctors' call for the continued availability of heroin. The arguments escalated with the teaching hospitals of London unanimously opposing the ban. Questions were raised in the Houses of Parliament and a loophole was found in the legal component of the Home Secretary's decision. It was shown that drug laws permitting control of manufacture to prevent heroin's improper use did not permit its total prohibition. Eventually it was decided that licences for the manufacture of heroin would be issued after the end of the year, prohibition of heroin in the UK never happened, and it resumed its place in the *British Pharmacopoeia* where it has stayed ever since after its narrow escape from being consigned to oblivion. This happened despite the fact that over the years, in 1978, 1987, and again in 1995, the United Nations Commission on Narcotic Drugs passed other resolutions urging governments to prohibit the use of heroin in humans.

In the UK, however, its qualities as a stronger analgesic with the beneficial side effect of detachment and euphoria are considered useful as a painkiller and anxiolytic. This is still considered a reason for its continued use in palliative care and for the treatment of severe pain such as that of myocardial ischaemia despite the introduction of synthetic opiate analgesics and the alternative morphine. In patients with terminal disease and those who are unable to swallow, parenteral opiates (given by subcutaneous infusion) are widely used to control pain. Morphine is relatively insoluble in water and it would be impossible to formulate it at a concentration appropriate for subcutaneous infusion. Diamorphine is however very soluble in water and can be used in high concentrations in small volumes in an infusion pump. It is derived from and is similar in structure to morphine but is two to three times stronger than morphine, is shorter-acting, and has a greater euphoriant effect.

Outside the UK alternative strategies are used. Since the use of morphine is limited by its solubility hydromorphone is used in some countries. Fentanyl, a potent opiate used widely in anaesthetic practice, is available in the UK as an injection, or for administration as a transdermal patch, but its effects are often difficult to predict and fine dosage adjustments are more cumbersome and complicated to achieve. These drugs are no less dangerous than diamorphine to an individual in overdose or when given by a fast intravenous injection. Today heroin is mostly manufactured by MacFarlane Smith Ltd in the UK. In the last few years the annual amount of diamorphine manufactured for medical purposes (excluding treatment of addiction) has been around 300 kg. For the year 2000, in excess of 3400 kg of street heroin was seized by the police and customs and this in turn is a fraction of the amount in circulation at any one time.

Concerning the use of heroin for pain associated with cancer, the World Health Organization (WHO 2007) produces comprehensive guidelines for the relief of cancer pain which have been updated from time to time. The WHO also has an extensive network of individuals, centres, and organizations which tackle the problem of cancer pain on a global scale.

Interestingly there are wide disparities in the use of analgesics in different countries. In terms of individual consumption, the average per-capita consumption of morphine in 1998 in the 10 countries with the highest consumption levels was 31 g per 1000 inhabitants. In the 10 countries with the next highest consumption levels, the corresponding figure was 16 g per 1000 inhabitants. In the next 60 countries with a total morphine consumption of more than 1 kg, it was only 2 g per 1000 inhabitants. In the remaining 120 countries there was little or no morphine consumption with several African countries reporting no morphine consumption at all.

In many countries the pattern of use of controlled drugs is changing. Examples of this from the USA show a rapid rise in the use of oxycodone, morphine, and hydromorphone and a very steep increase in the use of fentanyl between 1990 and 1996 (Nicholson et al. 2003).

Heroin has two main methods of administration: injection into a vein or muscle or inhalation. The effects are similar but injecting the drug has an almost immediate and more concentrated effect. Subjective effects include euphoria, calm, and detachment with the associated removal of concerns or awareness of anxieties. Sedation and drowsiness are invariable and dose-related, continuing into sleep and coma if tolerance is low or the dose is more than that to which the individual is tolerant. Further effects include respiratory depression, asphyxia, and death depending upon these factors.

Important features of any opiate use are tolerance, dependence (both physical and psychological), and withdrawal.

Morphine has many brands (MST, MXL, Sevredol, Oramorph, and others) with differing rates or durations of action. Prepared for quick onset in those with acute pain or for long action in the control of ongoing pain in, for example, those with cancer, these drugs are all morphine preparations with similar effects. Morphine is the standard against which all other opioid analgesics are compared. It remains the most valuable analgesic for severe pain although it frequently causes nausea and vomiting and about 15% of patients are intolerant to it, experiencing severe side effects.

Morphine is frequently taken by people who obtain pharmaceutical preparations through misrepresentation or from sources diverted from proper supplies. It can be taken by mouth or injected. Its effects resemble those of heroin or other opiates and its addiction and tolerance potential are similar. It has in some places become a useful alternative to methadone as a substitute for heroin (Kraigher 2005).

Burprenorphine (Suboxone, Subutex) has been available in smaller doses than those used for the treatment of drug dependency for many years. It is used as an analgesic for all sorts of serious musculoskeletal and neuropathic pains. Its introduction in a sublingual format in recent years has been a significant addition to methadone as a drug for use in treatment of opiate dependency. Recent guidelines from the UK National Institute for Health and Clinical Excellence (NICE 2007a) compared its efficacy with methadone. It was concluded that it had a comparable value for the treatment of opiate dependency but with some limitations due to its preparation and diversion potential. Nevertheless its recent licensing in the USA for drug-dependency treatment, under strictly controlled conditions, makes it the first drug to be approved for this indication for many years (DATA 2000). Its increasing use in Europe, particularly France, has come at a time when treatment services in many countries have been expanding rapidly and when enthusiasm for engaging drug users in treatment has grown exponentially. Buprenorphine has been particularly popular among community treatment agencies where its stigma has been seen by patients to be less than methadone. Buprenorphine is an interesting opiate which has a double effect described as agonist and antagonist. This is different from other opiates as it has a morphine-like effect and an antagonistic quality which may cause withdrawal effects in patients dependent on other opiates. It has a much longer duration of action than morphine and sublingually can have a painkilling effect lasting 6–8 h. It is used as a painkiller in relatively small doses of 200–400 µg or as a treatment for opiate dependence in larger daily or several times a week doses. In recent years it has become a major therapeutic agent in the treatment of opiate dependence. In France and in Northern Ireland, for example, it is the principal drug prescribed for the treatment of opiate-dependence syndrome. Both these countries were for different reasons relatively late in initiating opiate substitute treatment for those dependent on heroin. The choice of an alternative to methadone was therefore available from the start and may have been seen as an alternative associated with less hazardous side effects. Whether or not this is true remains to be seen. Buprenorphine has, in many other countries, become a useful addition to the more widely used methadone and is sometimes preferred by patients for this treatment.

Methadone

Methadone is a synthetic opiate pharmaceutically prepared originally in Germany in the 1930s. It is a drug which is prescribed for the treatment of pain and for the treatment of opiate dependency. In its former role it is an effective treatment in the management of chronic pain, often for those receiving palliative care for incurable illness. Its benefit derives from its opiate activity and, in particular, its long action in the body. For the treatment of opiate dependency it is extremely effective in long-term management of opiate-dependent patients, acting as a substitute for illegal and more damaging drugs such as heroin and morphine. Equally importantly it provides a legal alternative to a lifestyle complicated by all the dangers consequent on using a drug which is not prepared properly for consumption and which draws users into contact with an illegal underground as well as the criminal justice and law enforcement establishment.

Methadone is, therefore, widely prescribed by doctors and nurses and, inevitably, used inappropriately when it is diverted from proper sources to be used outside medical supervision. It therefore causes considerable damage in the form of addiction in those not previously addicted and overdoses in those unaccustomed to it.

As there are now estimated to be several million drug injectors in the world, and a much larger number of heroin users who do not inject, methadone is a widely prescribed medication. Despite is undoubted efficacy and potential life-saving properties it remains controversial and in some countries it is a banned substance. In Russia at present methadone is banned despite an epidemic of HIV infection in injecting drug users and similar epidemics of HIV infection are at present unfolding in many Eastern and African countries (Mathers et al. 2008, Csete et al. 2009).

Other opiates such as hydromorphone, dipianone, pethidine, oxycodone, and tramadol are important as they are all widely prescribed in different countries either on their own or in combination with other painkillers. They all have abuse potential and are associated with familiar problems in different countries where they are more available. Oxycodone for example is widely available in small doses over the counter in the USA and is widely abused in the same way as codeine products are in the UK.

Cocaine, amphetamine, and other 'psycho stimulants'

What are psycho stimulants? The following descriptions and definitions come from the publication *Psycho Stimulants: a Practical Guide*, published by the Effectiveness Intervention Unit for the Scottish Government (2002).

Psycho stimulants are substances that excite the central nervous system. They have the potential to produce feelings of alertness and well-being. There are a whole host of naturally occurring psycho stimulants including caffeine, nicotine, ephedrine, and cocaine. However, there are also synthetic psycho stimulants, which are principally amphetamines.

Cocaine (coke, Charlie, snow) refers to cocaine hydrochloride, a white powder that is water soluble. It is usually taken nasally or by injection. **Crack cocaine** (rock) refers to cocaine alkaloid. It is purer and more concentrated than cocaine and is absorbed into the body faster than cocaine. It is not water soluble and is usually inhaled after heating, usually in a pipe.

Cocaine is derived from the coca plant which grows in South America, South-east Asia, Africa, and the West Indies. Coca has been used in South America for centuries as a stimulant and a cure for a variety of physical ailments. It has at times in history been considered to have important spiritual qualities and the Incas considered its use to be associated with high social status. Cocaine was isolated in the mid-nineteenth century and has a much more powerful and potentially damaging effect than the much milder coca. Cocaine is a stimulant like the amphetamines and ecstasy. It is used in medicine as a local anaesthetic or pain blocker. It is taken by nasal inhalation which can cause irritation to the mucous membranes and often leads to strong psychological dependency. Although its use in the UK has been slower to develop than in the Americas it is increasingly popular and available. It is still associated with the media, glamour, and fashion industries although it is often injected by those who use a variety of opiates and other drugs. It was, and is, popular in the USA in combination with heroin.

Amphetamines (speed, whizz): there are three basic types of synthetic amphetamine (laevoamphetamine, dextroamphetamine, and methylamphetamine). The most widely available is usually a powder containing the first two of these types. It can be snorted, dabbed from finger to mouth, or injected. Smoking is not common. Amphetamines have an interesting pedigree. They were used extensively as a stimulant during the Second World War and were reputed to be used excessively by the Japanese air force to keep active pilots awake. During the 1950s and 1960s these drugs were experimented with by a range of people as an adjunct to studying although evidence of the ineffectual nature of the learning while under the influence of amphetamines curtailed their use. More recently amphetamines have been a popular and available recreational drug. Their availability through synthesis from easily available precursors avoids the problems of international trade and transport. Side effects include agitation, confusion, and psychotic manifestations in behaviour as well as withdrawal symptoms. When taken by injection the damage associated with this form of administration is a feature. Amphetamine use was popular in Sweden in the 1960s and a crisis of mismanagement in government has been an important historical background to the present severe approach to drug legislation in that country.

Ecstasy (methylenedioxymethamphetamine, MDMA) is an important, fairly recent, addition to the psycho stimulant range of drugs of use and misuse. Originally synthesized approximately 100 years ago, it was used experimentally by therapists and doctors in patients with psychological problems. Its widespread used, however, exploded in the 1990s when in conjunction with the dance and 'rave' culture it became a common and very widely used drug at social events. This continues despite official disapproval, highlighted by the drug being made a Class A drug under the Misuse of Drugs Act in 2000. Concerns were concentrated after the widely publicized death of a young woman in the UK and anxiety spread rapidly about the alleged dangers of the drug. Its properties as a depleting agent of serotonin in the brain gave a theoretical backing to the belief that it might have long-term consequences in the form of serious depressive illness in users or former users. This link has yet to be formally established, as is the small amount of evidence to associate ecstasy with a psychiatric abnormality characterized by an anxiety state with very specific and localized features.

Users of ecstasy experience a positive euphoria and elation with a feeling of confidence and well-being. Side effects, to which serious problems such as collapse, seizures, and coma are attributed, are associated with dehydration which may be due to excessive activity (dancing), sweating in enclosed rooms, and raised body temperature.

Codeine and codeine derivatives such as dihydrocodeine often are available as over-the-counter drugs either as single compounds or used in small quantities mixed with drugs such as paracetamol or ibuprofen for the treatment of pain or inflammation. They are therefore available in a very large number of proprietary and branded formats. Despite being controlled drugs their availability without a prescription is due to the relatively low strength of the compound in each tablet. This leads the user to take large numbers of tablets in order to achieve a psychoactive effect. The extent of use and addiction to these drugs is essentially unknown and difficult to measure.

LSD (lysergic acid diethylamide) is a synthetic hallucinogenic drug first produced in 1938. Most drug users have tried it but it remains unpopular today after a brief period of experimentation in the 1960s and 1970s when it was used by young people experimenting with lifestyle drugs and by occasional experimental psychiatrists. Its powerful and often disturbing effects led to its use being controversial and claims of its properties as mind-expanding and spiritual are often recognized as unpredictable and destructive and more likely to cause mental instability than to have any beneficial characteristic. Other hallucinogens in traditional use are derived from plants such as the mescalin mushroom and the peyote cactus.

Benzodiazepines (diazepam, chlordiazepoxide, nitrazepam, temazepam, and others) are a group of drugs most of which are controlled in Schedule 4 of the Misuse of Drugs Act 1971 although temazepam was put into Schedule 3 some years ago after a upsurge in its abuse and in particular its abuse by injection. This group of drugs is extremely widely used in medicine from short-acting anaesthetic properties to treatment of insomnia, anxiety, and stress. Chlordiazepoxide is particularly widely used in the treatment of alcohol withdrawal and diazepam is used to terminate convulsions caused by epilepsy. The differences in actions depend upon their varying half life. Diazepam has a longer action than temazepam and therefore is used for sustained action rather than the shorter value of temazepam useful in getting people to sleep at night. Nitrazepam was previously used as night sedation but its longer half life makes morning tiredness a less desirable effect. In general the shorter-acting benzodiazepines have a greater addiction potential and have become less widely prescribed. This has led to a reduction in availability and consequent abuse of drugs such as lorazepam and lormetazepam. Benzodiazepines such as flunitrazepam (Rohypnol) and triazolam (Halcion) achieved notoriety as date-rape drugs (the former) and injected sedatives (the latter) and have been removed from formularies in several European countries. Abuse of those drugs widely prescribed is common. Injecting of this group of drugs is not generally favoured due to the rapid sedation that results but oral use is endemic and serious. Tolerance is easily achieved and excessive doses are sometimes taken. Addiction is common and long-term use frequent. Withdrawals are prolonged and characterized by agitation, insomnia, and vivid dreams; withdrawal seizures are reported but are not as common as sometimes suggested.

Major tranquillizers such as chlorpromazine, promazine, clozapine, haloperidol, resperidone, sulpiride, and others are a group of drugs which are not commonly favoured as drugs of misuse or recreational drugs as they have serious depressant effects. They are more appropriately known as antipsychotic or neuroleptic drugs which are largely prescribed in the treatment of psychotic disorders such as schizophrenia. Their tranquillizing effects are of secondary importance and their use is largely reserved for mania, brain damage, schizophrenia, toxic delirium, or agitated depression. In the short term they are sometimes used for severe anxiety. Abuse potential is present and sometimes drugs are used after being diverted from the original patient.

Side effects are common and include sedation, skin reactions, liver damage, and many others but the most troublesome side effects are extrapyramidal disorders in the form of a Parkinson-type syndrome with stiffness (dystonia), abnormal movements (dyskinesia), restlessness (akathisia), and a distressing rhythmic involuntary movement of the face, jaw, and tongue (tardive dykinesia).

Barbiturates (Nembutal, Seconal, Tuinal, Amytal) are a group of sedative drugs which have disappeared from view in non-specialist medical practice and also from street use over the last three decades. Despite their continued use in anaesthetic practice as critically important inducers of sleep and sedation and in the treatment of epilepsy, their removal from the general pharmacopeia came after a sustained campaign by the British Medical Association to eliminate their use from everyday practice. This was as a result of widespread abuse by the public and the identification of serious side effects. These detrimental effects were noted by national committees studying the range of drugs being misused by young people in the 1960s and included sudden death from overdosage, convulsion and seizures, and addictive dependence. The transfer of use to the benzodiazepines as an alternative drug for the treatment of insomnia and restlessness allowed for the virtual abandonment of barbiturates by prescribers.

Mandrax (methaqualone) is a drug which, like the barbiturates, has disappeared from use by the medical profession and consequently by those who would abuse it. Still available in countries outside Europe and sometimes identified as a contaminant of illegal heroin, it is a sedative drug with dependency potential.

Khat is a green-leafed shrub that has been chewed for centuries by people who live in the Horn of Africa and Arabian Peninsula. Its use has recently been noticed in Europe, including the UK, particularly among emigrants and refugees from countries such as Somalia, Ethiopia, and the Yemen. Khat is imported and sold at greengrocers in areas such as East London. It remains potent only for a few days and is strongest when fresh leaves are chewed. It can also be made into a tea or chewable paste. The khat plant itself is not controlled under the Misuse of Drugs Act 1971, but the active ingredients, cathinone and cathine, are Class C drugs. Cathininone may not be lawfully possessed or supplied except under a licence for research, although cathine may be prescribed. It is controlled by law in countries such as the USA, Canada, Norway, and Sweden. References to khat use can be found in Arab journals from the thirteenth century. Physicians prescribed khat to treat depression and lack of energy. The stimulant effects also mean it has been commonly used by peasants working long hours. In some Muslim countries where alcohol is banned, khat is commonly used in social situations, although khat is often condemned on religious and cultural grounds.

Khat is a stimulant drug with effects similar to amphetamine. Chewing it makes people feel more alert and talkative and suppresses the appetite, although users describe an ensuing calming effect when used over a few hours. Regular use may lead to insomnia (inability to sleep), anorexia, and anxiety. In some cases it may make people feel more irritable and angry and possibly violent. Psychological dependence can result from regular use so that users feel depressed and low unless they keep taking it. There has been concern about the use of khat and its effect on some of its regular users in the Somali community. While khat may be causing some problems for refugees from the war in Somalia its use needs to be viewed alongside the poverty and racism experienced by many of these people (DrugScope 2008).

Cannabis is an important and widely used recreational drug. Recent investigations into its status as a drug causing damage have improved understanding of its widespread availability and popularity as well as its effects (Advisory Council on the Misuse of Drugs 2002, 2006, Royal Society for the Encouragement of Arts, Manufactures and Commerce 2007). Its status as a drug causing harm has increased somewhat since an extensive review of the literature and a debate about its various effects. Cannabis undoubtedly is a powerful drug with effects which encourage its use, including psychological and physical dependency. Its positive effects include euphoria, a feeling of tranquillity, sedation, and detachment. Common adverse effects are agitation and panic, dependency, and mental health instability. Whether or not it induces schizophrenia in individuals who would otherwise not develop that condition is fiercely debated. It certainly can cause a psychotic reaction or illness which appears to be related—like alcohol which can cause similar effects—to the amount taken, with larger intake with stronger derivatives being more likely to cause this form of damage.

Cannabis is usually smoked in a cigarette with tobacco but can be inhaled through a cooling pipe device or ingested in a form made palatable by mixing it into a cookie or biscuit. The form most commonly seen in the UK is a resin block but increasingly the home-grown herbal leaf format is available. Other forms of cannabis depend on the country of origin and method of cultivation and preparation.

There is a significant lobby to increase cannabis availability as a drug to treat nausea (a preparation is available in the UK), insomnia, and multiple sclerosis (a debilitating and progressive neurological disorder with distressing effects). Beneficial effects include musculoskeletal as well as sedative and psychological ones. Problems remain, however, in proving its benefit over other drugs in clinical trials and governments are reluctant to license this drug when there are alternatives and no unique benefit has been demonstrated. During recent years there as been a marked increase in the proportion of cannabis smoked in the stronger form known as skunk. This increase is considered further in Chapter 3.

Ketamine has been a Class C drug since 2006 under the Misuse of Drugs Act 1971. It has been used for many years as an anaesthetic agent in hospital medicine but a few years ago became popular in the dance and rave scene rather like ecstasy. It is a stimulant causing hallucinations and euphoria like

LSD and in larger doses causes out-of-body experiences, dissociation, and lack of coordination. Tolerance develops quickly and psychological dependence, flashbacks, loss of concentration and attention, and psychosis are reported in prolonged use. In combination with other drugs and alcohol side effects are worse and more dangerous.

Gammahydroxybutrate (GHB, or liquid ecstasy) and **gammabutyrolactone** (GBL) are closely related drugs with anaesthetic and sedative effects. In the UK (Misuse of Drugs Act 1971) GHB has been a Class C drug since 2003. GBL was made a Class C drug in January 2010. GBL converts into GHB when the substance is ingested. GHB and GBL produce essentially the same effects. Both drugs are depressants which slow down body actions. Small doses may feel like having a few alcoholic drinks. Inhibitions can be lowered and libido increased. At higher doses they may cause sleepiness, nausea, vomiting, muscle stiffness, and confusion and can lead to convulsions, coma, and respiratory collapse. Combining the drugs with alcohol can be fatal (DrugScope 2010).

Mephedrone is a stimulant drug which has emerged on the so-called legal highs market. The drug is not currently controlled under the Misuse of Drugs Act. Effects include euphoria, alertness, talkativeness, and feelings of empathy. However, users can also become anxious or paranoid and the drug's stimulant properties risk over-stimulation of the heart (DrugScope 2010).

Solvent abuse (glue sniffing, volatile substance abuse) is common. Past reported use may occur in up to 10% of young people in some areas and in small numbers in others. A number of compounds are used as solvents in glues, paints, nail-varnish removers, dry-cleaning fluids, and degreasing compounds. Others are used as propellant gases in aerosols and fire extinguishers or as fuels such as petrol or cigarette lighter gas (butane). Most households, factories, and offices use a range of solvents which can be sniffed. Sniffing of anaesthetic agents and ether as well as nitrous oxide has been reported for many years by anyone who has access to these compounds, including the medical profession. Restrictions on the availability of glues and solvents and the increasing popularity of ecstasy in young people may have accounted for the decrease in use of volatile substances since a peak in use during the 1960s and 1970s.

Effects are similar to alcohol or sedating agents and intoxication is dependent on the amount consumed. Confusion, hallucinations, and accidents are all reported and death from suffocation, inhalation of vomit in the severely intoxicated, and even from the toxic effects of the gas or fluid on the cardiovascular system are possible. Tolerance occurs but true addiction with withdrawal features is less common and long-term damage is related to lifestyle and self neglect as well as associated drugs of misuse.

Phencyclidine (PCP, angel dust) is usually illegally manufactured in laboratories and sold as tablets, capsules, or coloured powder. It can be snorted, smoked, or eaten. Developed in the 1950s as an intravenous anaesthetic, PCP was never approved for human use because of problems during clinical studies, including intensely negative psychological effects. Like LSD and ketamine, phencyclidine can cause dissociative effects and profound psychological upset.

There are many other products and naturally occurring substances which have been used to induce a euphoric or intoxicated state. Mushrooms, peyote cactus, and other vegetable derivatives are taken by many people throughout the world. The need to find an intoxicant transcends cultures and time. Some drugs create more problems and induce worse damage than others and, as suggested above, other factors such as the mode of use, the presence of contaminants, and legal status can exacerbate the damage done. Problems can be of a medical, social, or a criminal justice nature and many experience a combination of all three. Many of these collateral problems will be considered in subsequent chapters.

The challenge for legislators, parliamentarians, and public health officials is to understand and to correctly categorize drugs and as a result derive and implement appropriate penalties and constraints on the improper use and supply of these dangerous substances. This has, however, to be in the context of what is currently acceptable and culturally normal in different countries and communities. A balance is required which needs to be constantly adjusted and redefined—not an easy task. The possibility of conflict between researchers, and politicians and other opinion leaders has been obvious for some time. The conflict has recently flared up into unprecedented hostility and conflict. This has international, as well as purely national, implications for the relationship between science and policy formulation. This theme is considered in greater detail in later chapters.

Chapter 3

Drugs: patterns of use

...I do not readily believe that any man, having tasted
the divine luxuries of opium, will afterwards descend
to the gross and mortal enjoyments of alcohol.
(De Quincey 1821, reprinted 1995, p. 3)

As outlined in Chapter 1, drug use in the British Isles has a long history. This chapter will present details of changes of drug use, especially since the emergence of the 'drug scene' among teenagers and young adults in the 1960s. This review will outline demographic and geographical variations and the upsurge in drug use (including polydrug use, the use of a variety of illicit and legal substances) among both men and women. It will feature the authors' own research indicating that the levels of teenage drug use in the UK were among the highest in Europe. This chapter will describe the adoption of new types of drug, such as ecstasy (MDMA), crack cocaine, 'skunk', cannabis, gammahydroxybutyrate (GHB), and mephedrone. It features the latest findings of the 2007 European School Survey Project on Alcohol and other Drugs (ESPAD). This unique study is eliciting detailed information about illicit drugs use as well as alcohol and tobacco use, among a sample of over 2100 teenage school students throughout the UK. It will be argued that illicit drug use has become firmly normalized throughout the UK.

As indicated in Chapter 1, the lands that comprise the UK have long been populated by highly drug-oriented people. This chapter provides an overview of the changes in patterns of illicit drug use in the UK during the past century. It must be acknowledged that although a vast amount of material about drug use exists, much of this is anecdotal and some of the 'evidence' is inaccurate or based upon prejudice rather than fact. Moreover, the idea of conducting formal 'research' into the nature and extent of both legal and illicit drug use is a relatively recent phenomenon. In fact the contemporary drug scene really emerged during the 1960s. This process coincided with and was part of the development of a distinctive youth culture in many countries, including the UK. Much has been written about this culture and its hedonistic, counter-cultural values.

The latter were exemplified by the slogan 'Tune in, turn on, drop out'. As already noted, some drugs such as cannabis and opium have extremely long histories for recreational and medical, religious, and other purposes. The development of derivatives of opium (morphine and heroin), coca (cocaine), and a host of completely new drugs fed humanity's curiosity and search for new sources of pleasure or enlightenment. Some people were excited and delighted by the advent of new drugs, while others were alarmed or appalled by them. It should be emphasized that the drug scene has both national and international aspects. Drugs, drug fashions, drug news, and discussion of drugs travel quickly, especially since the advent of the Internet and broadband. In fact the drug scene began to blossom in an age of highly developed mass media: radio, television, magazines, books, drug-oriented music, and fashions. Young people in Europe were virtually as free to access the writings of Timothy Leary and other drug 'gurus' as were their counterparts in North America. Today, most aspects of illicit drug use are globalized (Alexander 2008).

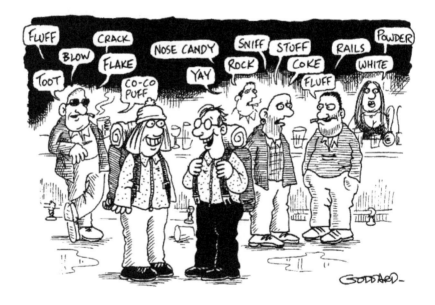

"Apparently, the locals have over 40 different words for snow!"
Credit: Cartoon Stock.com

The British drug scene, with its cannabis culture and associated use of other substances, was preceded by a rather different phenomenon, in the form of recreational amphetamine use by young people in the 1950s. This behaviour was not obviously associated with much of a philosophy, far less with any intellectual or spiritual aspirations.

Becoming a drug user

Most illicit drug use occurs within a social setting. This is because before a person uses a substance such as cannabis, it is necessary to decide to use it and to be able to obtain it. Most people begin to use drugs of some kind after they form friendly relationships with existing users. These generally provide them with their first experience of drug use. Moreover, they also demonstrate how to use the drug and, in some cases, teach novices how to appreciate the effects of the drug. This process has been described by Becker (1953–1954) in his classic work 'Becoming a marihuana user'. In fact first drug use is generally preceded by a process of reassurance and encouragement to experiment. This may well involve 'neutralizing' any prior reluctance or misgivings. Young people often report that their families are hostile to drug use. Many studies have examined how people generally begin to use drugs. These indicate that drug initiation usually takes place in a convivial setting and that most people are introduced to their first drug by people whom they know, rather than by strangers who are selling drugs (Goode 1970, 1972). Initial fears and reservations are allayed by friendly and reassuring contact with likeable people who already use drugs. This contact is likely to be accompanied by a degree of encouragement to try a drug (most commonly cannabis). Initial use is usually prompted by the observation that the existing users enjoy smoking cannabis and appear to be unharmed by this activity (Matza 1964, 1969, Plant 1975).

Studies of UK teenagers show that almost all of those who have used drugs report being introduced to them by either friends or older siblings. Often first drug use had involved a group of friends sharing the experience. Moreover, teenagers often report that they can obtain cannabis in places such as school, bars, in the street, in a park, or from the house of a drug dealer (Hibell et al. 2000, 2004, 2009). Young people often recall their first drug experiences as being prompted by curiosity about drug effects, to get high or feel good, to join in with friends, to be cool, or in some cases for a dare. Young people who have refused the offer of drugs attribute this to reasons such as not wanting to take drugs, regarding drugs as wrong and fear of drug effects or addiction (Fuller 2008).

In fact the distinction between user and suppliers is blurred since many drug users buy and sell drugs. There are of course large-scale professional drug dealers, but these are remote from most users. Why do people use illicit drugs, especially in view of the fact that a considerable amount of information about them is not positive? Again, the most powerful factor in drug initiation appears to be contact with 'credible' people who use drugs and who commend their use and allay any fears about the drug. Such advocacy, even if very informal and brief, is a commonplace first step towards trying cannabis or other drugs. Drug use also depends upon availability, so the range of available substances is likely to vary at different times in specific settings. Once an individual has used a drug, they may decide that once is enough, or they may use again. Their choice is likely to reflect whether or not they enjoyed the drug effects and the ethos of drug use. Thereafter an individual's drug-use career may be influenced by many factors, notably their social relationships and choice of lifestyle.

Drug surveys

An invaluable insight into the nature and extent of illicit drug use is provided by surveys of self-reported use. Like surveys related to other behaviours such as drinking and smoking, or sexual behaviour, drug surveys have limitations. Firstly, survey coverage is often selective and quite limited. Most UK surveys have been related to specific groups of people (notably school and college/university students). Survey coverage is almost always incomplete because of refusals, non-contacts, and response bias (exaggeration or denial) (Aquilino and Losciuto 1990, Gfroerer et al. 1997). Caetano has stated that some researchers have been complacent about such problems. In recent years rates of response to surveys have been declining. This is at least partly because drug surveys are no longer the novelty that they once were, so fewer people consent to participate if invited to do so. Some survey subjects under-report, while others exaggerate. Some do this deliberately, while others simply cannot recall exact details, especially of distant events or those experienced while under the influence of alcohol or other substances. Moreover, people who take part in surveys are likely to differ from those who do not (Petzel et al. 1973, Smith 1995, Dillman 2000, Caetano 2001).

Evidence about bias due to the fact that some of the intended subjects do not participate is mixed. Some reports suggest that non-respondents may not differ much from those people who do participate (Crawford 1987, Lemmens et al. 1988, Caetano 2001, Cull et al. 2005). Other studies have produced contrasting conclusions. Leung and Yu (2006), for example, report that bias due to non-response was 'not negligible' in relation to reporting of psychoactive substance use. Lahaut et al. (2002) have concluded that abstainers were over-represented among survey non-respondents. Clearly, it is wise to treat survey results with a degree of caution. Inaccurate results can be especially misleading in relation to unusual behaviours (such as the use of a rare drug when even a 1% or 2% error can hugely inflate or reduce evidence of prevalence). In spite of their likely limitations, surveys have enabled us to build up a general (if inevitably partial and imprecise) picture of which groups of people have used which drugs.

Drug use across the UK

The recreational use of cannabis and other illicit drugs in Britain, though it did occur, appears to have been rare before the 1960s (Plant 1975, Edwards and Busch 1981). Since then it is clear that drug use has increased to such an extent that many people, especially teenagers and young adults, view at least the use of cannabis as normal and socially acceptable. By the 1960s and 1970s a number of studies showed that substantial numbers of students and other young adults (e.g. 'hippies', young middle-class professionals, and bikers) had integrated cannabis in particular into their lifestyles (Binnie and Murdock 1969, Hindmarch 1970, Plant 1975). Cannabis was often adopted as a symbol of more general social attitudes and as part of a rejection of 'traditional' values (Young 1971).

Adolescents, school students, and college and university students

A 1979–1980 survey of 15–16-year-old school students in the Edinburgh area revealed that 7% of both males and females reported having used cannabis (Plant et al. 1985). A 1986–1987 survey of secondary school and college students aged 11–19 in Portsmouth and Havant indicated that 4% of respondents had at some time used cannabis. The proportions who had done so rose from none among the youngest respondents to 5% among those aged 14–15 and 11% among those aged 16–19 (Brown and Lawton 1988). A survey of London young people aged 11–16 indicated that 12% had used cannabis (Swadi 1988). Parker et al. (1987) surveyed self-reported drug use among 15–16-year-olds in schools in the Wirral during 1986. This indicated that a far higher percentage, 36%, had used this drug than had been evident in the Hampshire study by Brown and Lawton. Loretto (1996) surveyed 1172 secondary school students aged 14–16 in Scotland and Northern Ireland in 1992 and 1993. This study indicated that levels of cannabis use were higher in Scotland (46.2% of males and 33.1% of females) than in Northern Ireland (36.6% of males and 28.2% of females).

Most surveys of illicit drug use have been conducted in largely urban areas. Dean (1990) concluded from a qualitative study of adolescents in the Western Isles of Scotland that illicit drug use, especially that of cannabis, was 'widespread but not universal'. During 1994 a survey examined the use of cannabis and other psychoactive substances among 804 teenagers in schools in the

Western Isles. This showed that 34.6% males and 18.1% of females surveyed, most of whom were aged 14 and 15, had used cannabis. Forty-three per cent of the males who had used cannabis had done so on five or more occasions, whereas 50.8% of female users had tried the drug only once. Use increased with age and this study also showed that the use of cannabis and other drugs was associated with the heavier use of alcohol and tobacco (Anderson and Plant 1996). A series of studies monitored levels of drug knowledge and experience among secondary school students in three Wolverhampton schools between 1969 and 1994. These did not inquire into drug use itself. Even so, they have provided an invaluable guide in relation to a number of important issues. The 1994 study showed that over the 25-year period the proportion of students who knew someone who had used illicit drugs more than quadrupled, while the proportion who had been offered drugs increased more than nine-fold. Both proportions more than doubled between 1989 and 1994. Cannabis was the most commonly mentioned drug in the 1994 survey (Wright and Pearl 1995).

Surveys of Youth Training Scheme (YTS) and college students in the Wirrall were conducted in 1985 and 1986. These showed that 32% and 39% respectively had used cannabis. Almost all of the YTS students were male (Parker et al. 1988). These authors further concluded that 'regular' drug use among such individuals typically involved either using only cannabis, or cannabis and one other substance. Webb et al. (1996) carried out a survey of over 3000 second year students from 10 UK universities. This indicated that over 50% had used cannabis at least once.

More recently a study of medical students at the University of Newcastle-upon-Tyne concluded that over two-thirds had used cannabis (Newbury-Birch et al. 2001).

Other surveys

Most of the original study group of Edinburgh secondary school students surveyed in 1979 and 1980 were surveyed again, aged 19–20. The proportions who had used cannabis had risen considerably from 7% for both sexes to 22% of females and 35% of males (Plant et al. 1985).

A study of 162 offshore oil- and gas-rig workers used urine analysis for cannabinoids. This showed that 9.2% tested positive (Calder and Ramsay 1987). A survey of random samples of surgical, psychiatric, and medical nurses in the Lothian Region elicited information from 597 individuals. This indicated that 18.5% of females and 34% of males had used cannabis, but not in the past 6 months. Five per cent of females and 13.8% of males had used this drug in the past 6 months (Plant, Plant and Foster 1991).

National surveys

During 1989 a survey of 11 080 students aged 9–15 years in 475 schools in England were surveyed by Rudat et al. (1992b). This study showed that 3% of girls and 4% of boys had used cannabis. The level of use increased with age and among respondents aged 13–15 this rose from 2% to 14% for girls and from 3% to 16% for boys. Cannabis use was more common among teenagers from an Afro-Caribbean background (5%) than among white teenagers (4%) or those from an Asian background (1%). Levels of cannabis use varied some-what by region. This study showed that the highest levels of cannabis use were evident in London and south-east England. Otherwise, there was only slight variation in other areas (Rudat et al. 1992b).

A Welsh survey obtained information from 2239 15–16-year-olds in secondary schools during 1990. This showed that 14.1% of females and 17.9% of males surveyed had at some time used cannabis (Smith and Nutbeam 1992). A recent study conducted in Belfast indicated that cocaine had reportedly been used by 3.8% of 13–14-year-olds and 7.5% of those aged 15–16 years (McCrystal and Percy 2009).

Cannabis is now widely used by teenagers and young people from all types of background. Even so, there is some evidence to support the conclu-sion that the use of this drug is particularly commonplace among teenagers who are not living with both parents. This view was supported by the Welsh survey of Smith and Nutbeam (1992) and more recently by Miller and Plant (1996). Miller (1997) concluded that it made little difference to this relationship whether the mother, the father, or both parents were absent. He further noted that the influence of family structure was either reduced or eradicated if four other factors were taken into account. These were the extent of psychological symptoms, social support, the degree of involvement in hobbies, and the degree of indulging in activities such as '…going out with friends, aggression and delinquency'. Miller (1997) theorized that teenagers living with both parents may be more family- and home-centred and that this might at least partly explain their reduced involvement with cannabis or other illicit drugs.

An invaluable series of surveys has examined legal and illicit drug use among national samples of 11–15-year-old school students in England. This series commenced in 1982 and was originally confined to tobacco, but questions about alcohol were added in 1988 (Fuller 2008). Illicit drug use was only included in the series in 1998. The 2008 study indicated the following:

> The prevalence of drug use has declined since 2001. In 2008, 22% of pupils said they had ever used drugs, 15% had taken any drugs in the last year and 8% had taken drugs

in the last month. In 2001, the corresponding proportions were 29%, 20% and 12%. Pupils were most likely to have taken cannabis (9.0% in the last year, down from 13.4% in 2001). 5.0% of pupils had sniffed glue, gas or other volatile substances in the last year and 2.9% had sniffed poppers. Other drugs asked about had been taken by less than 2% of pupils in the last year. Overall, 3.6% of pupils had taken any Class A drugs in the last year; this has remained at a similar level since 2001.

The proportion of pupils who have taken drugs increases with age. As in previous years, boys and girls are equally likely to have taken drugs in the last year, but boys are more likely than girls to have taken drugs in the last month. In 2008, 33% of pupils reported that they had ever been offered drugs, a decrease from 42% in 2001.

Recent drug use is associated with regular smoking and recent drinking. Pupils who have been excluded also have an increased likelihood of recent drug use compared with pupils who have not, and drug use is also higher among pupils who have truanted from school compared with those who had not.

(Jotangia and Thompson 2009, p.125)

The downward trend in illicit drug use between 2001 and 2008 is shown in Figure 3.1: Figure 3.2 provides additional details of trends in the use of cannabis, glues and solvents, and poppers by school students over the same period.

The invaluable British Crime Survey (BCS) provides information about the proportion of 16–59-year-olds and 16–24-year-olds reporting having used any drug ever, last year, and last month by gender. This is shown in Figure 3.3: The same survey also indicated the proportion of 16–59-year-olds who reported use of the most prevalent drug types in the last year (1996–2006/7) (Roe and Man 2006). This is shown in Figure 3.4.

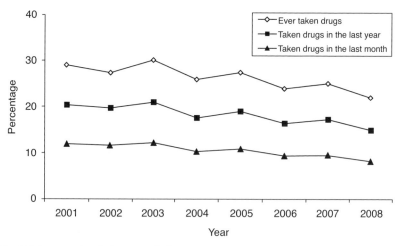

Fig. 3.1 Drugs taken in last month, last year, or ever, 2001–8.
Source: Copyright © 2010, Re-used with the permission of the Health and Social Care Centre. All rights reserved.

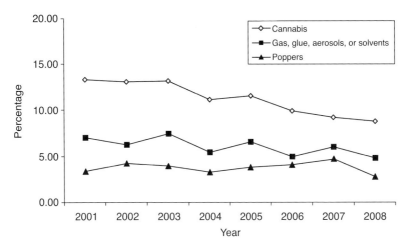

Fig. 3.2 Whether pupils had taken cannabis, solvents, and poppers in the last year, 2001–8.
Source: Jotangia and Thompson (2009).

General population

The Wootton Report (Advisory Committee on Drug Dependence 1968) estimated that 30 000–300 000 people in Britain had used cannabis. A BBC survey cited by Gossop (2007) suggested that 4 000 000 people had done so. Two market-research studies were conducted in 1979 and 1982. The first of these indicated that 12% of

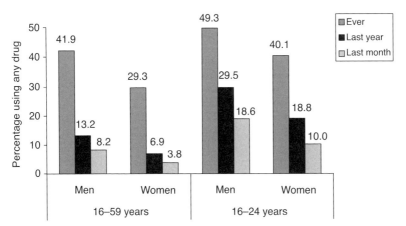

Fig. 3.3 Percentage of 16–59-year-olds and 16–24-year-olds reporting having used any drug ever, last year, and last month by gender, 2006–7 British Crime Survey (BCS).
Source: Murphy and Roe (2007).

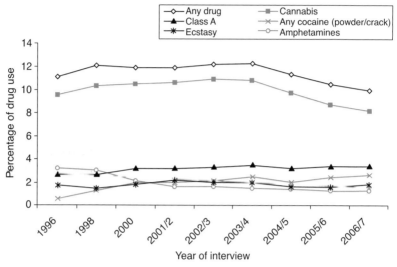

Fig. 3.4 Percentage of 16–59-year-olds reporting use of most prevalent drug types in the last year, 1996 to 2006–7.
Source: Murphy and Roe (2007).

those surveyed, 16% of males and 7% of females, had used cannabis. Cannabis use was higher among those who lived in the south of Britain (14%) than among those in the north (9%) (MORI 1979). This study related to a 'representative' general population sample selected by quota survey. The second study, also based upon a national quota sample, related to those aged 15–21. This showed that 17% of respondents had used cannabis. The latter survey found that cannabis use was especially high among the unemployed (27%), while this drug had been used by 10% of those in education and 17% of those in employment. This study lent further support for the conclusion that there were considerable regional variations in cannabis use. This ranged from 13% in south-east England, 15% in the north of England, 16% in the Midlands, East Anglia, and Wales, 21% in Scotland to 28% in London (NOP Market Research Ltd 1982).

The use of cannabis has become entrenched and, in effect, 'normalized' among many groups in British society beyond those who used it in the 1960s and 1970s (MacGregor 1989, Department of Health 1998, Parker et al. 1998, Hughes et al. 2001):

> People who use cannabis are not to be seen in terms of a single identikit picture- they are not all hippies, all Rastafarians, or all young executives. All general population studies have shown that most of those who have used cannabis have done so only a few times or have stopped.

> (Royal College of Psychiatrists 1987, p.127)

A similar journalistic view has been provided by James (1993):

> Unlike any other drug, marijuana is becoming an integral part of everyday living for not just the privileged few, the cultural makers and shakers, but whole sections of society from bricklayers to doctors, secretaries to soldiers.

> (p.30)

The British Crime Survey

The British Crime Survey (BCS) is a large-scale study of a representative sample of adults aged between 16 and 59 years residing in England and Wales. The BCS is a household survey. This probably provides a good picture of the most common forms of illicit drug use among household residents. Even so, it does not include all potential groups of drug users, notably those who are homeless or those living in institutions, including prisons and educational establishments.

> Nor, in practice, will any household survey necessarily reach those problematic drug users whose lives are so busy or chaotic that they are hardly ever at home or are unable to take part in an interview. As a result the BCS is likely to underestimate the overall use of drugs such as opiates and crack cocaine, covered by the survey.

> (Hoare and Flatley 2008, p.1)

The BCS has included a number of comparable questions related to drug use since 1996. These provide a valuable indication of drug-use trends since that year. There has been some variation in the questions included. Ketamine was considered for the first time in 2006/7. The BCS provides an indication of illicit drug use among people aged 16–59 years in England and Wales.

The BCS carried out in 1981 concluded that 16% of those aged 20–24 in England and Wales had used cannabis. The corresponding proportion in Scotland was slightly higher, at 19% (Chambers and Tombs 1984, Mott 1985). In 1995 a survey of 5020 people in 483 sampling areas in England was carried out. Respondents were aged 11–35. A total of 4932 individuals answered what were described as the most sensitive questions related to drug use. A substantial minority of the latter, 37% (or 36% of the total sample), had at some time used cannabis (BMRB International Ltd 1995).

The BCS (2000) found that between 15 and 28% of people in different parts of Britain who were aged 16–29 had used cannabis. The proportion of those aged 16–24 in England and Wales who had used this drug was 26%. A total of 13% of English 11–15-year-olds and 26% of 16–24-year-olds had used cannabis in the past year. Overall, drug use was found not to have increased between 1994 and 2000 (Ramsay et al. 2001, Department of Health/Office for National Statistics 2002).

A report of findings from the 2002/3 surveys indicated that:

+ of all 16–59-year-olds, 12% had taken an illicit drug and 3% had used a Class A drug in the last year;

+ cannabis is the most frequently used drug: 3 million 16–59-year-olds had used it in the last year (11%);

+ people aged between 16 and 24 years are more likely than older people to have used drugs in the last year;

+ levels of drug use among 20–24-year-olds are higher than among 16–19-year-olds;

+ the majority of people using drugs in the last year had only used one type of drug.

(Hoare 2009)

According to the BCS 2005/6 self-completion survey:

+ 10.5% of 16–59-year-olds had taken an illicit drug in the last year;

+ 3.4% of this age group had used at least one Class A drug in the last year;

+ cannabis is the most frequently used drug, with 8.7% of 16–59-year-olds having used it in the last year;

+ compared to 2004/5, the figures for 2005/6 show a stable pattern for most Class A drugs;

+ Class A drug use among young people has remained stable between 1998 and 2005/6.

(Hoare 2009)

An excellent and very detailed overview of patterns and trends in drug use as shown by the BCS has been provided by Roe and Man (2006). These authors report that 34.9% of those aged 16–59 years in England and Wales had ever used illicit drugs, while 10.5% had done so in the past year, and 6.3% had done so in the previous month. The corresponding proportions of those who had used Class A drugs (such as ecstasy, LSD, heroin, cocaine, and crack) were 13.9%, 3.4%, and 1.6%.

Roe and Man report that illicit drug use is most commonplace amongst young adults:

> The younger (16 to 19 and 20 to 24) age groups reported higher levels of more recent (last year and last month) drug use than the older age groups, while the high level of lifetime use amongst the 25 to 29 and 30 to 34 year old age groups is due to relatively high levels of use in the past. In particular: The 20 to 24 and 25 to 29 age groups reported the highest levels of lifetime use of any drug in 2005/06 (49.0% and 51.6% respectively), while the 30 to 34 age group reported greater lifetime use of any drug

compared to the 16 to 19 age group (45.8% compared to 40.4%). The 16 to 19 and 20 to 24 age groups reported the highest levels of last year use (24.8% and 25.6%) and last month use (14.6% and 15.5%) of any drug.

(Roe and Man 2006, p.21)

Like many other authors, Roe and Man note that males are more likely than females to have used illicit drugs. This difference is shown in Figure 3.3. The figure presents an overview of trends in drug use among this age group between 1998 and the 2006/7 BCS.

Trends in any illicit drug use

Between 1998 and 2005/06, the use of any illicit drug in the past year decreased from 12.1% to 10.5% of 16 to 59 year olds. The decline in any illicit drug use reflects the decrease in cannabis use, which has fallen from 10.3% in 1998 to 8.7% in 2005/06 due to significant year-on-year decreases since 2003/04…

Between 2004/05 and 2005/06 the use of any illicit drug in the past year declined, reflecting the further decrease in the use of cannabis.

Trends in Class A drug use

Compared with 1998, Class A drug use in the past year among 16 to 59 year olds in 2005/06 has increased from 2.7% to 3:4%. Between 2000 and 2005/06 the use of Class A drugs has remained stable.

The increase in Class A drug use since 1998 is mainly due to an increase in last year cocaine powder use from 1.2% in 1998 to 2.4% in 2005/06.

Between 1998 and 2005/06 the use of LSD decreased from 0.8% to 0.3% but the overall use of hallucinogens has been stable.

The use of ecstasy, crack cocaine and opiates has remained stable.

Compared to 2004/05, the figures for 2005/06 show a stable pattern for most Class A drugs, except for an increase in the use of cocaine powder in the past year…

Trends in use of other drugs

There have been some decreases among the 16–59-year-olds in the use of other drugs between 1998 and 2005/06, most notably a decrease in use of amphetamines (from 3.0% to 1.3%).

Additionally, there were decreases in the use of tranquilisers (from 0.7% to 0.4%), the use of steroids (from 0.3% to 0.1%) and use of glues (from 0.2% to 0.1%).

Between 2004/05 and 2005/06 the use of tranquilisers in the previous year continued to decrease.

(Roe and Man 2006, pp.12–13)

These trends are shown in Figure 3.4.

Roe and Man note the following levels of drug use reported in the previous year:

Consistent with previous years, cannabis is the drug most likely to be used. The 2005/6 BCS estimates that 8.7% of 16 to 59 year olds used cannabis in the last year… Cocaine is the next most commonly used drug with 2.4% claiming to have used any form of cocaine (either cocaine powder or crack cocaine) in the last year. This is followed by ecstasy at 1.6% and amphetamine use at 1.3%. Amyl nitrite use in the last year is estimated at 1.2% and use of hallucinogens (LSD and magic mushrooms) at 1.1%. Other drugs are very rarely used with only 0.4% reporting use of tranquillisers in the last year, 0.1% reporting use of anabolic steroids and 0.1% reporting use of glues. Other more serious drugs are also very rarely used: opiate (heroin and methadone) use was reported by 0.1% of 16 to 59 year olds.

(Roe and Man 2006, p.10)

More recent detailed information has been provided from the 2007/8 BCS (Hoare and Flatley 2008). This again covered a household sample of people aged 16–59 years living in England and Wales. The survey revealed that there had been a decline in self-reported drug use since the previous BCS in 2006/7. Overall the proportion of people who had used drugs in the past year fell from 10% to 9.3%. The previous year's use of cocaine, ecstasy, amphetamines, cannabis, and glues/solvents had dropped. The proportion of those who had used any Category A drug (such as heroin, cocaine, ecstasy, LSD, magic mushrooms, and methadone) fell from 3.4% to 3.0%. Overall, 35.8% of those surveyed reported having at some time used an illicit drug. Cannabis was by far the most common drug that had been used. A total of 7.4% had used it in the past year. Cocaine was the second most commonly used drug, which 2.3% reported having taken

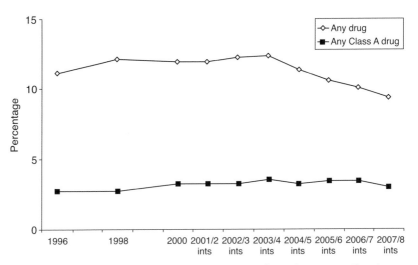

Fig. 3.5 Proportion of 16–59-year-olds reporting use of any drug or any Class A drug in the last year, 1996 to 2007–8.
Source: Hoare and Flatley (2008).

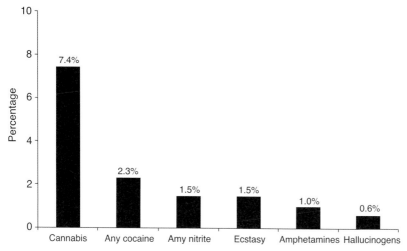

Fig. 3.6 Proportion of 16–59-year-olds reporting use of the most prevalent drugs in the last year, 2007–8.
Source: Hoare and Flatley (2008).

during the last year. The extent of illicit drug use is shown in Figure 3.5. The use of the most commonplace drugs is shown in Figure 3.6.

The BCS shows that illicit drug is extremely widespread. Hoare and Flatley (2008) have estimated that 11 467 000 people aged 16–59 years in England and Wales have at some time used illicit drugs. They also estimated that 4 469 000 people have used Category A substances. The BCS shows that the proportions of people aged 16–59 years who have used illicit drugs had declined since 1996. The proportions of those using Category A drugs has remained relatively stable. This is shown in Figure 3.5.

Hoare and Flatley reported that there had been a decline in drug use among younger BCS respondents, those aged 16–24 years:

> The use of any illicit drug by young people fell from 29.7% in 1996 (and 31.8% in 1998) to 21.3per cent in 2007/08… The longer-term decrease in young people's drug usage is in large part due to the gradual decline in cannabis use.

> (Hoare and Flatley 2008, p.21)

There had been a parallel reduction in the proportion of all 16–24-year-olds who were classified as being 'frequent drug users'. This had declined from 11.6% in 2002/3 to 7.3% in 2007/8. The authors also noted that: 'The apparent decline in the prevalence of young people's frequent drug use between 2006/07 and 2007/08 was not statistically significant'. The fall in the use of drugs, including Category A drugs, among younger adults is shown in Figure 3.7.

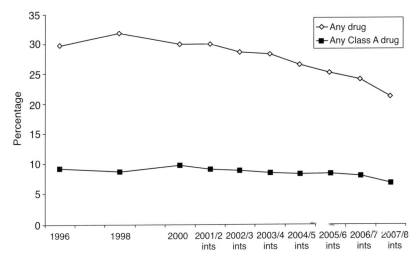

Fig. 3.7 Proportion of 16–24-year-olds reporting use of any drug or any Class A drug in the last year, 1996 to 2007–8.
Source: Hoare and Flatley (2008).

Additional information from the 2008/9 BCS has been provided by Hoare (2009). This report included the following summary of recent drug-use patterns and trends in England and Wales.

The 2008/9 BCS estimates that:

◆ Around one in three (36.8%) had ever used illicit drugs, one in ten had used drugs in the last year (10.1%) and around one in 20 (5.9%) had done so in the last month.

◆ Levels of Class A drug use were, unsurprisingly, lower than overall drug use, with 15.6 per cent having used a Class A drug at least once in their lifetime, 3.7 per cent having done so in the last year and 1.8 per cent in the last month.

◆ Consistent with previous findings, cannabis is the type of drug most likely to be used;
7.9 per cent of 16 to 59 year olds used cannabis in the last year.
The BCS has collected information on illicit drug use since 1996. Long-term trends for those aged 16 to 59 show:

◆ Use of any illicit drug in the last year has shown an overall decrease from 11.1 per cent in 1996 to 10.1 per cent in 2008/09, due in part to successive declines in the use of cannabis between 2003/04 and 2007/08.

◆ Despite this long-term overall decline, there has been an increase in last year use of Class A drugs among 16 to 59 year olds between 1996 (2.7%) and 2008/09 (3.7%). Usage has remained generally stable over this period: year-on-year changes were not statistically significant until most recently; however there was a slight underlying upward trend, which is now significant over the long term.

◆ The increase in Class A drug usage since 1996 can be understood in terms of an increase in last year cocaine powder use (from 0.6% to 3.0%), partly offset by a decrease over the same period in the use of LSD (from 1.0% to 0.2%). In 2008/09 methamphetamine was included for the first time but this has no visible impact on the overall prevalence of Class A drug use in that survey year.

♦ There have been some decreases over the longer term in the use of non-Class A drugs; between 1996 and 2008/09 last year use of cannabis, amphetamines and anabolic steroids among 16 to 59 year olds declined.

Changes between 2007/08 and 2008/09 showed:

♦ The overall level of any illicit drug use in the last year remained stable (9.6% in 2007/08 compared with 10.1% in 2008/09) but there was an increase in last year Class A drug use (from 3.0% to 3.7%).

♦ For individual types of drug, increases were seen in last year use of cocaine powder, ecstasy, tranquillisers, anabolic steroids and ketamine.

(Hoare 2009, p6)

Shaw et al. (2009) have provided a detailed review of statistical information related to drug use in England. This draws upon sources such as the BCS and the Office for National Statistics. They have reported the following conclusions.

> The lifetime rate of cocaine use has increased overall, and substantially in most English regions between 2002/03 and 2007/08, with the exception of London… Approximately 47,000 crack cocaine users are estimated to live in London (2006/07), resulting in a significantly higher rate per 1,000 population (aged 15–64) than the national average. The percentage of under 18s who reported use of any drug in the last year varied from 11.4% in the East of England to 19.6% in the South West.

(Shaw and Bellis 2009)

The most recent BCS figures indicate that cocaine use has risen from 1.3% to 6.6% between 1996 and 2009. The National Treatment Agency also reported that 3000 people aged between 18 and 24 had sought treatment for cocaine addiction in the past year (BBC News Online, 2 March, 2010b).

It should be noted that although the alleged adulteration of illicit drugs by dealers has periodically been widely publicized, often to scare people away from drug use, this practice has generally appeared to be rare. As noted by Coomber (1997a, 1997b, 1997c, 1997d, 1999) most of the illicit drugs in circulation in the UK appear not to have been adulterated. Even so, the fall in the use of cannabis and some other drugs should be set in the context of convincing evidence that there has recently been a substantial increase in the use of stronger 'skunk' cannabis or 'sinsemilla'. The potency of cannabis is determined by its content of delta-9-tetrahydrocannabinol (THC), the primary active constituent. It has been reported that while strong skunk accounted for only 15% of cannabis used in England and Wales in 2002, this proportion had risen to 75–80% by 2008. The use of milder cannabis resin, it was noted, had declined from 60–70% in 2002 to only 20% by 2008. This change has been attributed to the increased activity of Vietnamese drug dealers. The use of skunk has been linked with schizophrenia (Hope 2008).

The European Monitoring Centre for Drugs and Alcohol Addiction (EMCDDA 2008) has reported on the levels of purity of European heroin:

> In 2006, the typical purity of brown heroin ranged between 15% and 25% in most reporting countries, although values under 10% were reported in Greece, France and Austria, and higher ones in Malta (31%), Turkey (36%) and the UK (43%). The typical purity of white heroin was generally higher (45–70 %) in the few European countries reporting data.

> (EMCDDA 2008, p.70)

In fact some drug contamination does occur. This was tragically illustrated by the deaths of several drug users in parts of Scotland including Glasgow, Fife, and Lanarkshire in late 2009 and early 2010. These unfortunate individuals had apparently used heroin that had been contaminated with the deadly disease anthrax. It was speculated that the heroin in question had been 'cut' with animal bonemeal, possibly in a country (such as Afghanisthan or Turkey) where anthrax is more common than it is in Britain (McAulay and Duffy 2009, Carrell 2010).

The latest annual Street Drugs Trends survey by the charity DrugScope (2009a) did conclude that most drug prices were stable or had declined, but that there had been a downward trend in the quality of available drugs:

> This year's findings show a fall in the reported quality of illegal drugs available in most areas over the last year. Seventeen out of twenty areas reported a drop in the quality of powder and crack cocaine, echoing a growing body of evidence showing declining cocaine purities. In one area, police reported seizing cocaine powder with purity levels as low as 2%. Twelve out of the twenty areas reported a decline in heroin quality, while the majority of areas also highlighted a fall in the MDMA content in ecstasy pills and a continuation of the long-term trend in poor quality amphetamine.
>
> The fall in quality has also occurred in the illicit market in prescription tranquillisers, notably diazepam. While authentic 10mg pills diverted into the black market were being sold in most areas for £1, fake, low quality, versions reported to be from labs in China and South-east Asia were available for half the price in some areas.
>
> The survey found that the drop in the quality of drugs could be accelerating a longer term trend towards poly drug use–taking a variety of different substances in combination or at different times–as users look to 'top up' on low quality drugs or experiment with alternatives. In turn, some survey respondents suggested that the shift towards people using a more varied menu of drugs means users are less concerned about the quality of each individual substance.
>
> In some areas older teens and younger adult recreational users are swapping or combining substances including cocaine, ketamine, GHB/GBL, ecstasy, cannabis and alcohol. Problem drug users in most areas are often using heroin and crack cocaine alongside cheap, strong alcohol, skunk-like cannabis, tranquillisers and, in some cases, ketamine.

Survey respondents expressed concerns that the low quality of stimulants such as cocaine, crack, speed and ecstasy pills could be contributing to a growing interest in other substances. Ketamine, the hallucinogenic anaesthetic, was reported as being used by a growing number of older teens and young adults in 18 out of 20 areas surveyed. For the first time in the survey's five year history, some drug services raised concerns about the use of the so-called 'legal highs' GBL and mephedrone.

(DrugScope 2009a, p.1)

Northern Ireland

Invaluable information about drug use among people aged 16–59 years in Northern Ireland has been provided by the 2006/7 Northern Ireland Crime Survey (Ruddy and Brown 2007). As in England, this survey showed that cannabis was by far the most widely used illicit drug. Twenty per cent of respondents reported having used this drug at some time, and 6% had used it in the past year. The survey also concluded that the prevalence of past month's illicit drug use had declined from 6% in 2003/4 to 4% in 2006/7 (McMullan and Ruddy 2005). As indicated by other studies, the Northern Ireland Crime

Table 3.1 Last year's drug use in Northern Ireland (2006/7)

	All adults (%)	Males (%)	Females (%)	16–24 years (%)	25–34 years (%)	35–59 years (%)
Any drug	8.4	10.6	6.4	22.0	10.3	3.5
Amphetamine	0.5	0.8	0.2	1.4	0.6	0.2
Cannabis	6.3	7.9	4.7	17.8	8.6	1.8
Cocaine	0.9	1.5	0.4	2.0	2.1	0.2
Crack	*	0.1	0	0	0.2	0
Ecstasy	0.9	1.4	0.5	3.0	1.1	0.2
Heroin	0	0	0	0	0	0
LSD	0.1	0.1	0.2	0.2	0.2	0.1
Magic mushrooms	0.2	0.3	0.1	0.8	0	0.1
Methadone	*	0.1	0	0	0.2	0
Tranquillizers	0.5	0.8	0.3	0.6	1.3	0.3
Amyl nitrate	0.6	0.7	0.5	2.0	0.4	0.2
Steroids	0.3	0.6	0.1	1.2	0.2	0.1
Glues	0.1	0.2	0	0.6	0	0
Unweighted base (N)	2390	1103	1287	342	578	1470

*Less than 0.1%.

(*Source*: Ruddy and Brown 2007, p.5).

Survey indicated that the highest levels of drug use were evident among males and among people aged 16–24. This is elaborated in Table 3.1, which refers to the prevalence of the past year's drug use. As the table shows the self-reported use of drugs other than cannabis was low. Even among the most drug-oriented group, those aged 16–24, only ecstasy had been used by more than 2%. The use of opiates (heroin and methadone) as well as cocaine and crack was rare. It should of course be reiterated that surveys of this type may be biased by under-reporting. They may also fail to include the heaviest drug users.

Scotland

The Scottish Crime and Victimisation Survey (SCVS) (formerly known as the Scottish Crime Survey) provides an invaluable picture of self-reported drug use among 16–59-year-olds in Scotland. The most recent study in this series was conducted in 2006 (Brown and Bolling 2007). This survey, which had previously used paper questionnaires, employed Computer Assisted Personal Interviewing (CAPI) in 2006. This resulted in the reporting of higher levels of drug use than had been noted previously.

The 2006 survey indicated that 37% of those surveyed had used some kind of illicit drug at some time in their lives. A total of 17% of respondents reported having used a Category A drug. Thirteen per cent of those surveyed reported having used an illicit drug in the past year and 8% had done so in the past month. The authors concluded that:

> Although reported levels of lifetime drug use in Scotland were broadly similar to those reported in England and Wales in 2005/6 by the British Crime Survey (BCS), reported levels of current drug use were higher in Scotland compared with England and Wales, where 10% reported using drugs in the last year and 6% in the last month.

> (Brown and Bolling 2007, p.2)

It is well established that there are regional variations in tobacco smoking and alcohol consumption and rates of their associated problems (Crawford et al. 1984, Latcham et al. 1984, Balarajant and Yuen 1986, McAleney and McMahon 2006, Goddard 2006, Plant and Plant 2006). Alcohol consumption appears to be heaviest in the north of England. Alcohol-related morbidity is highest in the most deprived areas of Britain, in the West of Scotland, and in the least prosperous urban areas in England and Wales (Herald 2007). Smoking and its catastrophic ill effects on health are also most prevalent in the most deprived areas and among groups of people with the lowest socio-economic status.

The surveys described in this chapter make it clear that illicit drugs are used by people from a wide range of varied backgrounds. Even so, Roe and Man (2006) have also presented an interesting picture of the regional variations in drug use in England and Wales. Approximately 10% of those aged between 16 and 59 years in England and Wales reported having used illicit drugs in the past year. Roughly 3% reported the use of Class A drugs in this period. Total drug use was highest in the south-west of England, followed by the north-west and London. Class A drug use was highest in London. The regional variations were not great and are shown in Table 3.2.

A more recent picture of regional variations in England has been provided by the analysis by Shaw et al. (2009) of the 2007/8 BCS. This is shown in Table 3.3, which illustrates that rates of recent drug use were highest in south-west England, Yorkshire and Humberside, and north-west England. They were lowest in the West Midlands and eastern England.

It appears that there were only low levels of illicit drug use in Northern Ireland before the 1990s. This reflected many factors including the social disruption associated with 'the troubles'. The recent return to a more peaceful situation may involve the normalization of both nightlife and crime (McElrath 2004, Mc Ellrath 2009).

Drug testing

Some groups of people, such as air crew members, military personnel, and prisoners, are subjected to compulsory drug testing. Such testing in the workplace is not common, but has been increasing. Studies have indicated that the proportion of employers using such tests may be in the range of 4%–16%

Table 3.2 Percentage of 16–59-year-olds who had used drugs in the past year by Government Office Region (2005/6 BCS)

Region	Any drugs (%)	Class A drugs (%)
North east	9.8	3.7
North west	11.6	3.4
Yorkshire and Humberside	9.0	2.7
East Midlands	9.2	3.0
West Midlands	9.1	2.6
Eastern	10.3	3.2
London	11.2	5.2
South east	10.1	3.3
South west	13.3	3.2
Wales	10.2	2.8
England and Wales	10.5	3.4

(*Source*: Roe and Man 2006, pp.26–27).

Table 3.3 Rates per 1000 of population of people aged 15–64 in England who had used drugs in the past year

Region	Males	Females	Total
North east	103.45	63.41	82.59
North west	134.87	62.62	95.79
Yorkshire and Humberside	131.61	62.33	96.80
East Midlands	123.72	55.08	89.49
West Midlands	115.07	46.93	79.10
Eastern England	103.63	56.13	78.32
London	118.61	58.11	87.59
South east	120.67	50.83	82.98
South west	126.52	68.74	96.97
England	120.75	57.57	87.74

(*Source*: Shaw et al. 2009, p.53; figures from the North West Public Health Observatory, derived from the BCS (weighted).).

(Joseph Rowntree Foundation/DrugScope 2004). Recent evidence from the British Army (which tests 85% of its personnel annually) indicates that the use of illicit drugs among their workforce has been increasing.

> Research into Compulsory Drugs Testing (CDT) of UK service personnel, published today by the Journal of the Royal United Services Institute (RUSI), has identified a rise in positive tests for illegal substances in the British Army from 517 individual cases in 2003, to 795 in 2005 (and 769 in 2006), and also a four-fold growth in soldiers testing positive for the class-A drug cocaine.
>
> (Royal United Services Institute for Defence and Security Studies 2007; see also Bird 2007)

Mandatory drug testing in prisons in England and Wales was introduced in 1996. Reports relayed to this programme indicate that testing underestimates drug use. Singleton et al. (2005) concluded from a survey of prison inmates that 66% reported having used drugs in the month prior to incarceration. In contrast, only 25% reported having done so while in prison. In addition the Department of Transport has highlighted concerns about drug-impaired driving. There is currently no approved breathalyser-like device for use to measure such drug use.

During 2004 the then Prime Minister Tony Blair declared his support for the random drug testing of school students. This complex and sensitive issue has been reviewed by McKeganey (2005), who concluded that the evidence base to support the introduction of such a policy is weak. Moreover, he concluded, this might be both costly and damaging.

Polydrug use

It is evident that, while cannabis is by far the most widely used illicit drug, many people at some time also use other substances such as ecstasy (MDMA) or cocaine. In fact there is abundant evidence that people who are heavy drug users or who use a wide range of illicit drugs are commonly heavy drinkers and tobacco smokers. The distinguished American researcher Eric Goode once wrote the following:

> … people who use illegal drugs, marijuana (cannabis) especially, are fundamentally the same people who use alcohol and cigarettes- they are a little further along the same continuum. People who abstain from liquor and cigarettes are far less likely to use marijuana than people who smoke and drink.
>
> (Goode 1972, p.12)

In fact most of those who use cannabis do not use other illicit drugs. Most cannabis users do not take even this drug for prolonged periods or use it heavily when they do. Drug fashions change over time and the availability of specific substances varies too. Many studies have shown that individuals who are heavy users of legal and illicit drugs are also often inclined to engage in other 'risky' behaviours. These include having unprotected sex and driving without seat belts (Jessor and Jessor 1977, Hingson and Kenkel 2004). Numerous studies have concluded that both young people and adults who are heavier drinkers are also more likely to use other substances such as tobacco and illicit drugs (e.g. Goode 1969a, b, 1970, 1972, Plant 1975, Miller and Plant 2002, Hughes et al. 2008).

Heavy drug users are also those most at risk of experiencing adverse consequences from their drug use. The use of drugs is influenced by their price and availability (see Petry 2000, 2001). A recent analysis by Sumnall et al. (2004) concluded that among a group of British polydrug users, there was substitution of some drugs for others in response to price changes. Cocaine, for example, was used to substitute for ecstasy if the latter rose in price. Similarly alcohol was adopted as a substitute if amphetamine increased in price.

Stepping stones/escalation?

One of the traditional arguments against using cannabis and so-called 'soft' drugs such as amphetamines is that they are 'gateway' drugs or 'stepping stones' to 'harder' or more dangerous substances. The latter include heroin and cocaine. In fact this contention is both right and wrong. Firstly, the first psychoactive drugs that most people use are alcohol and tobacco, not cannabis. Secondly, as noted above, many cannabis users do not use other illicit drugs and most do not become heavy or long-term users. Thirdly, it is true, as

Goode has stated, that if an individual never uses cannabis (or alcohol or tobacco), he/she is less likely to use other drugs than would otherwise be the case. Accordingly, it is true that cannabis may be a gateway to other forms of drug use. This is because some cannabis users do take other drugs, have access to supplies of such substances and may commend their use.

User careers

Drug use is influenced by many factors. These include gender, socio-economic position, family influences, peer-group pressures, religion, nationality, region, occupation, income, education, age, life events, drug availability, and price. Drug use generally occurs in a social context, as already noted. Studies indicate that young people generally use legal substances before embarking on the use of illicit ones (Kandel 1978). Thereafter drug use often involves using cannabis or a limited number of other substances for a few years, then cutting down or ceasing drug use. This is exemplified by the many students who smoke cannabis while at college but seldom, if ever, do so later in life. It should be emphasized that by far the most widespread and pernicious chronic form of drug use from a health perspective is tobacco.

Heavy users

As already emphasized, there is an association between using illicit drugs and taking legal drugs. An examination of recent UK survey findings about drug use among teenagers led to rather inconsistent conclusions. An analysis of survey data elicited from 15- and 16-year-old school students in 2007 supported the following conclusion:

> The strongest predictor of teenage substance use was the age at which the first 'real drink' was consumed. Those who took their first drink before the age of nine years were the heaviest users as teenagers. Young people who had their initial drink later in life were lighter users of both legal and illicit drugs by the age of 15 and 16 years.

> (Plant and Miller 2008)

Findings from the same study were also examined to explore the possible association between early parental guidance related to drinking alcohol and later substance use. This revealed that the highest level of drug use was found among teenagers whose parents were more favourable towards alcohol, those who were also more tolerant of them getting drugs and also among teenagers who did not answer questions on this subject. The latter group were especially likely to have used cannabis and other illicit substances (Miller and Plant 2010).

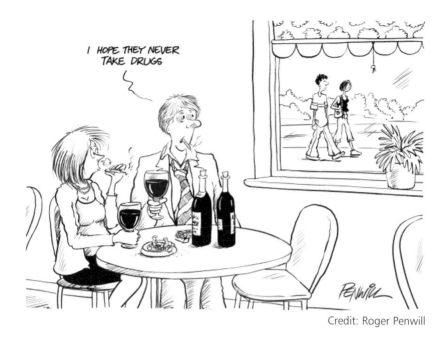

Credit: Roger Penwill

The lowest levels of drug use were evident among teenagers whose parents were restrictive in relation to their children consuming alcohol.

There is considerable evidence suggesting that young people who are the heaviest users of illicit drugs are especially likely to be raised in single-parent families. This is evident, both within the UK and in other countries (Miller 1997, Ledoux et al. 2002, Miller and Plant 2003a). It should be noted that in the UK single-parent families are often on low incomes and are frequently headed by an unemployed parent. A Swedish study showed that children who had been reared by single parents had significantly higher rates of alcohol and drug-related problems in adulthood than other people (Weitoft et al. 2003). In contrast, Velleman and Templeton (2003) have concluded that many such young people are far more resilient and are less affected by parental substance use than has often been acknowledged.

Even so, parents are very important. It seems that heavy involvement with legal and illicit drug use and other risky behaviours is associated with lack of parental support, supervision and control, and poor relationships with parents (Barnes and Farrell 1992, Swadi 1999, Miller and Plant 2003a, Robbins et al. 2008). It has been widely reported that children and young people who have been raised by adults who are heavy or problematic alcohol or drug users may also use such substances heavily later in life (Jessor and Jessor 1977, Plant and Plant 1992). The role of parents is given further consideration below.

The club scene

Since the spread of illicit drug use, it has been associated with music, leisure, and young people. The 'club scene' that developed in the UK in the 1980s was strongly associated with the use of ecstasy (Ashton 1992, Sherlock 1999, Parker and Williams 2001, Measham 2002, Riley and Hayward 2004, Hadfield and Measham 2009). In fact this drug was widely used at large-scale raves, some of which were attended by thousands of dancers. One police officer remarked to one of the authors that the use of ecstasy at a rave was far less likely to result in disorder than the consumption of alcohol. The appeal of illicit drugs in the context of dancing was alleged to prompt some producers of alcoholic beverages to adopt drug-related styles and images to promote their products. Drug (including alcohol) fashions change over time. The club scene inevitably reflects such changes, with variations in the types and quantities of substances (such as cocaine and nitrous oxide ('laughing gas')) that are available and in vogue with clubbers (Kirby 2006). A survey of drug use among a non-representative group of 1000 readers of the *Western Eye*, the student newspaper of the University of the West of England, Bristol, indicated that 10% of those who responded had used laughing gas (*Western Eye* editorial staff, personal communication).

A study by Hutton (2004, 2006) indicated that nightclubs vary considerably. Moreover, she concluded that some clubs enable women to develop a 'positive feminity' that is distinctive from the traditional, more passive, female social role.

Drug use in international perspective

Illicit drug use occurs on a huge international scale. The United Nations World Drug Report for 2005 estimated that approximately 200 million people had used such substances in the previous year. It was also acknowledged that approximately 30% of all adults smoked tobacco and that half consumed beverage alcohol (United Nations Office on Drugs and Crime 2005). The United Nations (2009) has recently noted that the worldwide numbers of drug users had grown to an estimated 4343 million people aged 15–64 years who had taken drugs at least once in the past year during 2007. These included 11–21 million intravenous drug users and 18–38 million 'problem drug users'. The United Nations has further reported that:

> The year 2008 saw some encouraging reductions in the production of cocaine and heroin. In cooperation with the affected states, UNODC [United Nations Office on Drugs and Crime] conducts annual crop surveys in the countries that produce the vast

bulk of these drugs. These surveys show a reduction in opium poppy cultivation in Afghanistan of 19% and a reduction in coca cultivation in Colombia of 18%. Trends in other production countries are mixed, but are not large enough to offset the declines in these two major producers.

Although data are not complete enough to give a precise estimate of the global reduction in opium and coca production, there can be little doubt that it did, in fact, decrease.

Production of the other illicit drugs is more difficult to track, and data on drug use are also limited. But surveys of users in the world's biggest markets for cannabis, cocaine and opiates suggest these markets are shrinking.

According to recent surveys of young people in Western Europe, North America, and Oceania, cannabis use appears to be declining in these regions. Data from the world's biggest cocaine consuming region, North America, show a decrease, and the European market appears to be stabilizing. Reports from traditional opium-using countries in South-east Asia also suggest the use of this drug may be declining there. Heroin use in Western Europe appears to be stable.

In contrast, there are several indications that the global problem with amphetamine-type stimulants (ATS) is worsening. Global seizures are increasing, and ATS are being made in a growing number of countries, with diversifying locations and manufacture techniques.

Close to 30% of global seizures in 2007 were made in the Near and Middle East, where amphetamine use may also be significant. Methamphetamine precursors are increasingly being trafficked to Central and South America to manufacture ATS for the North American market, and local use also appears to be going up. The size of the ATS market is large, and likely still growing in East Asia. Data on ATS are particularly problematic, however, and UNODC is making a concerted effort to improve monitoring of trends in this area.

Of course, all these markets are clandestine, and tracking changes requires the use of a variety of estimation techniques. Data are sparse, particularly in the developing world, and the level of uncertainty in many matters is high.

(United Nations Office on Drugs and Crime 2009a, p.9)

The levels of illicit drug use in the UK are high by international standards. Useful information on comparative levels of illicit drug use are available from the EMCDDA and the World Health Organization (WHO). The EMCDDA (2008) has reported that it is evident that the level of drug use in Europe has been stabilizing and that in some countries it has declined. The EMCDDA has recently reported that the prevalence of illicit drug use (and problematic opioid use) in Europe is as follows:

Cannabis

Lifetime prevalence: at least 71 million (22% of European adults)
Last year use: about 23 million European adults or one-third of lifetime users...

Cocaine

Lifetime prevalence: at least 12 million (3.6% of European adults)
Last year use: 4 million European adults or one-third of lifetime users...

Ecstasy

Lifetime prevalence: about 9.5 million (2.8% of European adults)
Last year use: over 2.6 million or one-third of lifetime users...

Amphetamines

Lifetime prevalence: almost 11 million (3.3% of European adults)
Last year use: around 2 million or one-fifth of lifetime users...

Opioids

Problem opioid use: between one and six cases per 1,000 adult population.

(EMCDDA 2008, p.13)

The EMCDDA (2008) also reports that the prevalence of illicit drugs in the UK is among the highest in Europe. This is exemplified by the fact that the highest levels of cannabis use among those aged 15–34 years are evident in Denmark (49.5%), France (43.6%), the UK (41.4%), and Spain (38.6%). Levels of amphetamines, LSD, ecstasy, cocaine, and crack cocaine were higher in the UK than in other European countries.

The European School Survey Project on Alcohol and other Drugs

An international perspective on teenage illicit drug use, drinking and smoking in the UK has been provided by the European School Survey Project on Alcohol and other Drugs, widely known as ESPAD. This large-scale investigation is described in more detail below. ESPAD has collected information from representative samples of 15- and 16-year-old school students in Europe. The first ESPAD survey in 1995 involved 29 countries. It showed that 44% of boys and 38% of girls in the UK had at some time used cannabis. Altogether 42% (44% of boys and 40% of girls) reported at some time having used an illicit drug. This was the highest level reported by teenagers in any of the 29 participating countries and was also marginally higher than in a comparable US study of teenagers (Grant and Dawson 1997, Hibell et al. 1997). In fact ESPAD showed that while cannabis was by far the most widely used drug among European teenagers, levels of illicit drug use varied greatly. These ranged from 40% in the UK to 9% or fewer in Croatia, Cyprus, Estonia, Finland, Hungary, Lithuania, Malta, Norway, Sweden, Poland, Portugal, and Turkey (Istanbul only). Only Ireland, where 37% of teenagers had used illicit drugs, reported a level of use approaching that in the UK. Altogether between 10% and 23% of teenagers in the Czech Republic, Italy, Denmark, Ukraine, Slovenia, the Faroe Islands, Iceland, and the Slovak Republic reported having used illicit drugs.

This initial ESPAD showed that teenage boys in the UK were significantly more likely to have used cannabis than were girls. Scottish teenagers were the highest cannabis users. Among females levels of cannabis use in the constituent parts of the UK were: 47.4% (Scotland), 38.0% (England), 31.4% (Wales), and 15.9% (Northern Ireland). The corresponding proportions among males were as follows: 59.8% (Scotland), 41.9% (England), 34.5% (Wales), and 34.9% (Northern Ireland). These results were consistent with the findings of Loretto (1996) that cannabis use and other illicit drug use was less commonplace in Northern Ireland than in Scotland (Miller and Plant 1996). Teenagers in the UK reported the highest level of experience of having used illicit drugs other than cannabis (22%). They also reported the highest level of consuming alcohol with 'pills' (20%). In many other European countries, levels of the last two behaviours were much lower. Taken overall, ESPAD showed that UK teenagers had much higher levels of illicit drug experience than those in most other European countries, apart from those in neighbouring Ireland.

ESPAD also showed that UK teenagers, together with the Irish, Danes, Italians, and Finns reported high levels of 'binge' (or 'risky single-occasion') drinking three or more times in the previous 30 days. A binge was defined for this study as having consumed five or more drinks on a single occasion. Teenagers in the UK were particularly likely to report having been drunk and experienced adverse effects from their drinking. This is elaborated in Chapter 4. ESPAD indicated that most European teenagers aged 15 and 16 years had tried tobacco. Teenagers in the Faroe Islands were those most likely to have smoked in the past 30 days (42%), followed by those in Ireland, Ukraine, Finland, and Turkey (Istanbul only), and the UK. A total of 40% of girls and 32% of boys in the UK reported having smoked tobacco in the past 30 days.

The second ESPAD survey in 1999 found that although UK school students still had the highest overall level of illicit drug use (36%) this was nearly equalled by teenagers in the Czech Republic and France (35%). A total of 39% of UK boys and 33% of UK girls reported having used some form of illicit drug, mainly cannabis. In comparison, contemporary US studies suggested that 41% of teenage high school students had used cannabis (compared with 35% in the UK, the Czech Republic, and France). This compared with 14% or less in Poland, Estonia, Bulgaria, Lithuania, Norway, Hungary, Finland, Greece, the former Yugoslav republic of Macedonia, Portugal, Sweden, the Faroe Islands, Malta, Cyprus, and Romania (Hibell et al. 2000).

The picture changed when the third ESPAD was carried out in 2003. This survey included teenagers from 35 European countries. The highest levels of illicit drug use were reported by school students in the Czech Republic (44%), Switzerland (41%), Ireland (40%), and the Isle of Man (40%). The UK and France ranked next (both with 38%). Levels of drug use reported by teenagers elsewhere ranged from over 30% in Belgium, Germany, and Spain to less than 10% in Cyprus, Greece, Norway, Romania, Sweden, and Turkey (Hibell et al. 2004).

ESPAD 2007

The most recent ESPAD was conducted in 2007. As noted above, this study had been conducted previously in 1995, 1999, and 2003 (Hibell et al. 1997, 2004, Smart and Ogborne 2000). Even so, it must be emphasized that ESPAD is a cross-sectional investigation, not a prospective study of a single group of respondents. The UK part of the 2007 survey took place from March until July in that year. It covered school students born in 1991 who were aged 15 or 16 during the survey. The sample covered schools in the UK as a whole, making no distinction between England, Scotland, Wales, and Northern Ireland. Limited resources (time and money) permitted coverage of 120 schools (including two classes from each school). Schools were sampled across the UK probability proportional to size and making no other distinctions. Participating schools then supplied a list of all their classes containing pupils born in 1991, and two of these classes were randomly sampled from these lists. The field work on these two classes was carried out by a designated teacher during the period March to July 2007. The standard ESPAD questionnaire was completed by students in each class under 'examination' conditions. Instructions to the students emphasized that each student had been chosen randomly, and that the answers were anonymous and totally confidential. It was also emphasized that participation was voluntary and that they need not respond to questions which they disliked.

Information was obtained from 2179 students (1004 boys and 1175 girls) aged 15 and 16 years attending 99 schools. Fieldwork was unexpectedly arduous and time-consuming. A total of 203 schools were sampled of which 117 agreed to participate. Ultimately, 18 of the latter disappointingly failed to take part. The final school response was disappointing, at 48.8%. This was lower than in previous phases of ESPAD. There were no detectable differences in the types of schools cooperating and not cooperating. It was evident that UK schools have been becoming increasingly resistant to participating in studies of this type (Fuller 2009b). The most common reasons given for school refusals was that the school had taken part in other research projects and the fact that staff or students were already greatly overloaded with commitments, including national Office for Standards in Education, Children's Services and Skills (Ofsted) inspections. The latter were clearly strongly disliked. They appeared to be a major cause of stress among teachers. Fortunately the response rate among students in schools that did take part in the survey remained as high as in past years, at 83.6%. Most non-participating students were either ill or absent with permission on the day of the survey in their class. ESPAD 2007 included the following 35 countries: Armenia, Austria, Belgium, Bulgaria, Croatia, Cyprus, the Czech Republic, Denmark, Estonia, Faroe Islands, Finland, France, Germany, Greece, Hungary, Iceland, Ireland, the Isle of Man, Italy, Latvia, Lithuania, Malta, Monaco, the Netherlands, Norway, Poland, Portugal, Romania, Russia, the Slovak Republic, Slovenia, Sweden, Switzerland, Ukraine, and the UK. Over 100 000 students participated in this exercise. An additional five countries also participated in 2008, but at the time of writing findings from these were not available.

Overall, there had been a decline in cigarette smoking among ESPAD students across Europe since the previous survey in 2003. Smoking had dropped by 4% between 1995 and 2007 in countries that had comparable data over this period. Lifetime prevalence of smoking across Europe ranged from 24% and 80%. Smoking in the past 30 days ranged from 7% in Armenia to 45% in Austria. Altogether 22% of UK teens (17% of boys and 25% of girls) had smoked in the past 30 days.

Lifetime illicit drug use among teenagers across Europe had risen between 1995 and 2003. It had fallen since then. Teenage drug use in the UK had fallen since 1995. The highest lifetime use of any illicit drug was reported by teenagers in the Czech Republic (46%), followed by Spain (38%) the Isle of Man (35%), and Switzerland (34%). UK teenagers ranked ninth out of 35 in this respect (29%). The lowest levels of drug use were evident among teenagers in Cyprus, the Faroe Islands, Norway, Romania, and Armenia (4%–7%). The highest lifetime use of cannabis was reported by teens in the Czech Republic (45%), Spain (36%), the Isle of Man (34%), and Switzerland (33%). UK teenagers ranked seventh in this respect (29%). A total of 11% of UK teenagers (13% of boys and 10% of girls) reported having used cannabis in the past 30 days. As in earlier ESPAD surveys, far fewer teenagers reported having used other drugs than had smoked cannabis. The self-reported lifetime levels of illicit cannabis use among girls and boys in the study countries in 2007 are shown in Figures 3.8 and 3.9.

The levels of other drug use ranged from none in Armenia to 16% in the Isle of Man. Altogether, 9% of both boys and girls in the UK reported having used some drug apart from cannabis. The use of glues and solvents ranged from 3% in Bulgaria, Lithuania, Spain, and Ukraine to 17% in the Isle of Man. Nine per cent of UK teenagers (10% of girls and 8% of boys) reported such use.

The use of tranquillizers and sedatives without prescription was also examined. The levels of such use ranged from none in Armenia and only 2% in the UK to 10%–16% in Poland, Lithuania, France, Monaco, and Italy.

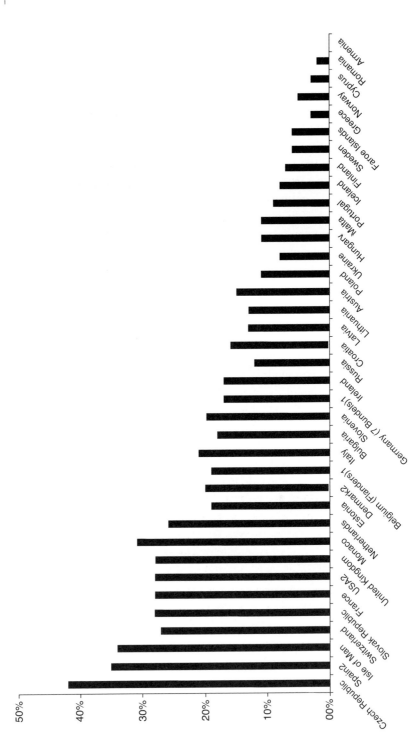

Fig. 3.8 ESPAD 2007: lifetime use of cannabis in females.

A 1 after a country means that only certain regions were surveyed; a 2 means limited comparability; because that country's data are not from ESPAD.

Source: Hibell et al. (2009).

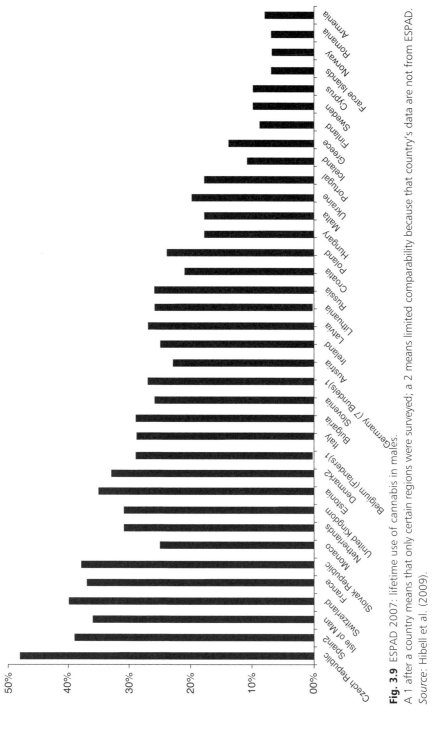

Fig. 3.9 ESPAD 2007: lifetime use of cannabis in males.

A 1 after a country means that only certain regions were surveyed; a 2 means limited comparability because that country's data are not from ESPAD.

Source: Hibell et al. (2009).

Teenagers were asked to indicate to what degree cannabis was easy to obtain. The European average was that 35% of boys and 31% of girls reported that it was 'fairly easy' or 'very easy' to get cannabis. UK teenagers were much more likely to respond in this way. Altogether 53% of boys and 48% of girls reported that cannabis was easy to obtain. Only teenagers in the Czech and Slovak Republics exceeded this level. Teenagers in the UK were also particularly likely to indicate that they thought it was easy to obtain ecstasy (18%) and glues and solvents (66%). In addition, 15% reported that it was easy to obtain tranquillizers or sedatives. Three per cent of UK teenagers reported having used ecstasy in the past year. In addition the lifetime use by UK teenagers of tranquillizers or sedatives without prescription was 2%. Lifetime use of other substances was: glues and solvents (9%), magic mushrooms (4%), GHB (1%), anabolic steroids (1%), drugs by injection (1%), and alcohol together with 'pills' (7%).

Consistent with previous ESPAD surveys, cannabis was by far the most commonly used illicit drug among those surveyed in 2007. The self-reported lifetime levels of cannabis among boys and girls in the study countries in 2007 are shown in Figures 3.8 and 3.9. Teenagers in the UK were ranked seventh in relation to cannabis use. Countries in which this was higher were the Czech Republic (45%), Spain (36%), the Isle of Man (34%), Switzerland (33%), the Slovak Republic (32%), and France (31%). A comparable US study had indicated a lifetime cannabis use rate of 31%. The corresponding UK rate was slightly lower at 29%. Among UK teenagers cannabis had been used by 30% of boys and 28% of girls. A total of 13% of UK boys and 10% of girls reported having used cannabis in the previous 30 days.

Overall, ESPAD 2007 indicated that UK teenagers were more likely than their peers in most but not all European countries to engage in binge drinking and to use illicit drugs. Even so they were not especially likely to smoke tobacco and relatively few had taken illicit substances other than cannabis. The non-prescription use of tranquillizers or sedatives appeared to be unusual. The ESPAD surveys showed that among UK teenagers, smoking and illicit drug use had declined between 1995 and 2007. Alcohol consumption (specifically 'binge drinking') remained above the European average and was relatively stable.

Another large-scale comparative international study, the Health Behaviour of School Children (HBSC) has examined a broad range of behaviours among secondary school students. Todd et al. (1999) have reported that the Scottish component of this investigation showed that illicit drug use had not changed among respondents aged 15 and 16 years between 1994 and 1998, apart from a rise in the percentage of girls who had tried cannabis. There had also been an increase in the proportion of 13-year-old girls who had used magic mushrooms in the past month.

Currie et al. (2008), reviewing HBSC findings, have noted that lifetime cannabis use among 15-year-olds in England, Scotland, and Wales in 2005/6 was as shown in Table 3.4. As this table indicates, regional differences in Britain were minor, although Welsh girls had slightly higher levels of use than Welsh boys. Welsh girls also reported higher levels of cannabis use than did their counterparts in England and Scotland.

The proportions of British 15-year-olds who had used cannabis within the last 30 days did not vary much in different regions. This is shown in Table 3.5.

The findings of the HBSC, like those of ESPAD 2007, showed that levels of cannabis use among British teenagers were high by international standards. Lifetime use was lower among school students in 29 European countries than in any part of Britain. Lifetime cannabis use was higher than in any part of Britain only in Switzerland.

Do parents matter?

The potential role of parents in relation to the drinking and smoking habits of their offspring are extremely important. As noted by Velleman (2009) family processes and structures may affect the knowledge, attitudes, and behaviour of young people. In addition, the peer group may influence both youthful legal and illicit drug use. The UK ESPAD questionnaire covered psychoactive substance use and gender, hobbies, family situation, parental educational level, parental monitoring, and relationships with peers and parents. Other optional sections used in the UK included parental attitudes, respondent's self-esteem, and level of depression. There has long been an active debate about the possible role of parents in influencing the use of legal and illicit drugs by their children. The family ethos is clearly one of the most important determinants of a child's psychoactive substance use (Velleman and Orford 1999, Ledoux et al. 2002, Miller and Plant 2003b, Engels et al. 2007, Järvinen and Room 2007) and there is some continuity between childhood and adult behaviour (Fillmore 1988,

Table 3.4 Lifetime cannabis use among 15-year-old school students in Britain

Country	Males (%)	Females (%)
England	26	23
Scotland	29	27
Wales	30	32

(*Source*: Currie C et al, eds. *Inequalities in young people's health. HSBC international report from the 2005/2006, survey*. Copenhagan, WHO Regional Office for Europe, 2008:136, 140 (http://www.euro. who.int/en/what-we-do/health-topics/Life-stages/child-and-adolescent-health/publications2/2011/ine-qualities-in-young-peoples-health).)

Table 3.5 Cannabis use in past 30 days among 15-year-old students in Britain

Country	Males (%)	Females (%)
England	10	8
Scotland	13	11
Wales	12	11

(*Source*: Currie C et al, eds. *Inequalities in young people's health. HSBC international report from the 2005/2006 survey.* Copenhagan, WHO Regional Office for Europe, 2008:136, 140 (http://www.euro.who.int/en/what-we-do/health-topics/Life-stages/child-and-adolescent-health/publications2/2011/inequalities-in-young-peoples-health).)

Dubow et al. 2008, Englund et al. 2008, Maggs et al. 2008, Merline et al. 2008, Schulenberg and Maggs 2008, Peck et al. 2008, Pitkänen et al. 2008, Zucker 2008). Parental attitudes and their consequences have been described by many authors (e.g. Barnes and Farrell 1992, Jackson et al. 1999, Mounts 2000, Ennett et al. 2001, Wood et al. 2004, Barnes 2005, Van Der Vorst et al. 2005a, 2005b, 2006). It has often been noted that in some countries, such as France and Italy, it has long been normal for children to be introduced to drinking by their parents and other family members (e.g. Heath 1995).

This has raised interest in the possibility that such early socialization into drinking might be a good approach to commend within the UK. Since drinking and other forms of drug use are often associated, this issue had relevance not only for drinking, but also for illicit drug use among teenagers. During the UK part of the 2003 ESPAD study teenagers were asked if they recalled having been taught to drink by their parents. Fewer than a fifth reported that this had been the case. Such teenagers were more likely than others to have drunk alcohol in moderate amounts on their last drinking occasion. Even so, there were no differences in the experience of alcohol-related problems or in the extent of binge drinking in the past 30 days. The taught group were slightly less likely to smoke cigarettes, but were not less likely than others to have used illicit drugs such as cannabis (Plant and Miller 2007).

The UK part of 2007 ESPAD included some additional questions related to the teenage students' memories of their first sip of alcohol ever and their first drink of at least one glass. This information could then be compared to other data collected in the survey concerning current psychoactive substance use.

One objective of this study was to examine the relationships between the types of parental guidance (if any) that teenagers had reportedly been provided with about drinking alcohol and teenage use of legal and illicit drugs. Statistical analysis indicated the following:

> Substance use was least common in the cluster in which parents strongly discouraged the use of alcohol and also, surprisingly, in the cluster where the respondents claimed to have been given no parental guidance at all. The highest substance users were found

firstly in students from families where there was a more favourable attitude to alcohol and a relative tolerance of getting drunk and secondly among students who failed to answer the questions on parental guidance. The latter in particular scored highly on the use of cannabis and other drugs. The cluster in which there was comprehensive discussion with the parents about all aspects of alcohol use had an intermediate position in relation to substance use. Thus being well-informed was not necessarily associated with abstinence or low level use. In logistic regressions parental guidance was consistently associated with substance use with several other background variables controlled.

(Miller and Plant 2010)

First drinks and teenage psychoactive substance use

An additional aim of the ESPAD 2007 study was to explore the possible association between teenagers' self-reported first drink and psychoactive substance use among respondents at the ages of 15 and 16 years. The investigation of this subject was supported by the Joseph Rowntree Foundation.

Methods

The focus of this analysis was parental guidance relating to alcohol and also the circumstances regarding the first sip and the first real drink of alcohol. The age at which the respondent had their first real drink was ascertained from a separate question. The parental guidance given was described in terms of seven clusters. Separate comparisons were first made between the first-drink variables and the rest using chi-square. Abstainers and those who failed to answer the questions concerning the first drink were excluded. Logistic regressions were then run between the substance-use variables and the first-drink variables using the stepwise forward logistic regression method and controlling for various demographic variables.

The survey was conducted between March and June 2007. Information was obtained from 2179 school students (1004 boys and 1175 girls) aged 15 and 16 years attending 99 UK schools. A total of 203 schools were sampled of which 117 agreed to participate. Ultimately, 18 of the latter failed to take part.

Abstainers and non-responders

A total of 220 respondents (10.1%) reported that they had never consumed alcoholic beverages. These abstainers comprised 101 boys and 119 girls and there was therefore no gender difference. Two hundred and seventy-five students (12.6%) failed to answer the relevant questions about the first drink. Both these groups of students are excluded from all the following analyses.

First drinking experiences and parental guidance

Where the parents' attitude to alcohol was relatively favourable the large majority of parents knew about the first real drink, the location was usually a 'safe' one (i.e. at home), and it most often happened below age 13. This may be contrasted to the cluster where the parents were very discouraging towards alcohol. In this cluster by far the lowest proportions of parents knew about the first drink, the location was significantly less likely to be a safe one, and the first real drink tended to take place later in life. Most students remembered their first experience of alcohol (i.e. even one sip), enjoyed the effect of their first real drink (at least one glass), and only a minority got drunk on the first real occasion. There were no significant differences between the clusters on these latter variables. (Note that significant means that a finding was unlikely to have occurred by chance. The significant test results noted in the following section are based upon the assumption that these was a 95% level of probability that findings were not due to chance.)

There was no relationship between the age of the first drink and getting drunk on the first occasion (chi-square 7.3, 6 degrees of freedom, not significant) but, if the student did get drunk on this occasion, the parents often did not know (17.8% knew, 48.8% did not know; chi-square 155.5, 2 degrees of freedom, $P<0.001$).

First drinking experiences and substance use

The results are shown in Tables 3.6, 3.7, and 3.8. Levels of statistical significance are shown, but should not be too confusing for most readers. Psychoactive drug use was not related to whether or not respondents (students) could recall tasting their first ever sip of alcohol. All the other first-drinking-experience variables showed highly significant relationships. For instance, if the parents did not know about the first real drink their offspring was significantly more likely to have been drunk more than five times in their lifetime, to have been binge drinking (consuming five or more drinks in a session) in the past 30 days, to have been seriously drunk on the last drinking occasion, to have smoked cigarettes, to have used cannabis, and to have used other drugs. There was a clear relationship between substance use and the age at which the first real drink occurred: the later the age the less the substance use.

Chi-square analyses were run to determine whether parental guidance affected the first drinking experiences. Students with controlling, restrictive parents were more likely than the rest to be substance users when their parents did not know about the first drink, when it was consumed in an unsafe

Table 3.6 Circumstances of the first drink and later alcohol use (%)

	Remembered the first ever drink		Fisher exact probability
	Yes N=1071	No N=585	
Got drunk more than five times in the lifetime	34.6	32.8	NS
Binge drinking at least once in the past 30 days	59.7	56.2	NS
Seriously drunk on the last drinking occasion	27.1	22.7	$P=0.052$
	Parents knew about the first real drink		
	Yes N=1191	No N=413	
Got drunk more than five times in the lifetime	30.7	45.3	$P<0.001$
Binge drinking at least once in the past 30 days	55.3	69.4	$P<0.001$
Seriously drunk on the last drinking occasion	22.2	37.5	$P<0.001$
	First real drink in a safe location		
	Yes N=1012	No N=620	
Got drunk more than five times in the lifetime	30.9	39.5	$P<0.001$
Binge drinking at least once in the past 30 days	53.8	66.6	$P<0.001$
Seriously drunk on the last drinking occasion	21.4	33.1	$P<0.001$
	Got drunk on the first real drinking occasion		
	Yes N=417	No N=1206	
Got drunk more than five times in the lifetime	60.2	25.5	$P<0.001$
Binge drinking at least once in the past 30 days	79.4	51.8	$P<0.001$
Seriously drunk on the last drinking occasion	47.4	18.4	$P<0.001$

(Continued)

Table 3.6 *(continued)* Circumstances of the first drink and later alcohol use (%)

	Enjoyed the effect on the first time		Fisher exact probability
	Yes N=1129	No N=459	
Got drunk more than five times in the lifetime	40.2	20.5	P<0.001
Binge drinking at least once in the past 30 days	66.3	41.1	P<0.001
Seriously drunk on the last drinking occasion	30.2	15.1	P<0.001

NS, not significant.

location, or when it happened before age 13. The results concerning parental knowledge and unsafe location broadly confirm this. For instance, when a student was in the 'discourage the use' cluster (controlling parents) and their parents did not know about the first drink, 55.3% had been drunk six or more times in their life. This is to be contrasted with the rest of the students whose parents did not know about the first drink, of whom only 31.8% had been drunk six or more times. The difference is significant. However, there is no such result when the first drink occurs before age 13. If anything the result is the other way round, but usually not significantly so.

Modelling substance use

Logistic regression models were explored predicting binge drinking in the past 30 days, daily cigarette smoking, lifetime cannabis use, and lifetime use of drugs other than cannabis. In addition to the first-drinking-experience variables the predictor variables selected were parental guidance, gender, parental education level, family financial position, self-esteem, depression, emotional support from friends, use of the Internet, going out in the evenings, frequently indulging in a hobby, and friends' substance use. Variables were entered stepwise using the likelihood ratio method. The results are given in Tables 3.9 and 3.10. After testing all the variables, current circumstances and behaviour remained strong predictors of substance use; for example, if most friends smoke the student is more than seven times as likely to be a daily smoker than if this is not true. If he/she goes out in the evening almost daily the odds ratio compared to those who go out almost never was 2.746. Having a hobby was found to be significantly protective against binge drinking and daily smoking, but not against other substance use. Associations were also found for depression or low self-esteem with binge drinking, smoking, and use of drugs

Table 3.7 Circumstances of the first drink, cigarette smoking, cannabis, and illicit drugs (%)

	Remembered the first ever drink		Fisher exact probability
	Yes N=1083	No N=589	
Ever smoked cigarettes	56.2	52.3	NS
Ever smoked cigarettes daily	22.7	19.3	NS
Ever used cannabis	30.3	28.8	NS
Ever used other illicit drugs	20.6	21.1	NS
	Parents knew about the first real drink		
	Yes N=1203	No N=418	
Ever smoked cigarettes	50.5	69.1	$P<0.001$
Ever smoked cigarettes daily	19.2	27.9	$P<0.001$
Ever used cannabis	25.6	43.1	$P<0.001$
Ever used other illicit drugs	18.2	28.2	$P<0.001$
	First real drink in a safe location		
	Yes N=1024	No N=625	
Ever smoked cigarettes	49.8	63.5	$P<0.001$
Ever smoked cigarettes daily	16.9	29.2	$P<0.001$
Ever used cannabis	23.6	40.6	$P<0.001$
Ever used other illicit drugs	17.5	26.3	$P<0.001$
	Got drunk on the first real drinking occasion		
	Yes N=423	No N=1217	
Ever smoked cigarettes	74.7	48.6	$P<0.001$
Ever smoked cigarettes daily	35.6	16.7	$P<0.001$
Ever used cannabis	50.0	23.4	$P<0.001$
Ever used other illicit drugs	34.5	16.1	$P<0.001$
	Enjoyed the effect on the first time		
	Yes N=1142	No N=463	
Ever smoked cigarettes	59.4	46.2	$P<0.001$
Ever smoked cigarettes daily	24.0	16.4	$P=0.001$
Ever used cannabis	34.8	20.0	$P<0.001$
Ever used other illicit drugs	24.0	14.0	$P<0.001$

NS, not significant.

Table 3.8 The age of the first drink and substance-use variables (%)

Age of first drink (years)	Substance-use variable (%)							Chi-square
	9 or less N=240	10 N=184	11 N=221	12 N=333	13 N=326	14 N=268	15+ N=137	
Got drunk more than five times in the lifetime	57.4	50.6	41.9	37.0	25.0	17.4	7.3	174.2***
Binge drinking at least once in the past 30 days	74.9	66.9	67.6	62.7	53.1	47.9	29.4	105.2***
Seriously drunk on the last drinking occasion	33.9	33.3	29.4	29.4	22.0	17.9	8.2	50.2***
Ever smoked cigarettes	71.0	66.3	63.8	56.9	48.5	44.2	27.9	99.9***
Ever smoked cigarettes daily	31.6	35.2	28.8	23.0	14.6	13.0	5.2	82.1***
Ever used cannabis	43.8	42.6	39.9	33.5	21.9	16.9	9.6	106.4***
Ever used other illicit drugs	37.5	35.3	24.9	21.9	13.2	6.7	6.6	127.9***

***$P<0.001$

other than cannabis. Females were more than twice as likely as males to be daily cigarette smokers.

However, after controlling for these variables, the circumstances surrounding the first drink still produced significant associations. In particular the age of the first drink was highly predictive. Compared to the 137 students who had their first real drink aged 15 or more, those 240 who had it aged 9 years or younger were 4.2 times as likely to have been binge drinking in the past 30 days, 6.1 times as likely to be daily cigarette smokers, 4.7 times as likely to have used cannabis, and 5.5 times as likely to have used other drugs. In general, getting drunk on the first occasion was predictive of all four dependent variables. An unsafe location for the first drink was associated with cigarette smoking and cannabis use. Enjoyment of the first drink was associated with binge drinking. Parents not knowing about the first drink was associated with cannabis use.

Many factors enter into the family ethos; for example, the emotional support the parents give their child, and the extent to which they seek to control their

Table 3.9 Logistic regression findings on binge drinking and daily cigarette smoking

	Five drinks in a row					
	Cox and Snell R^2=0.25, Nagelkerke R^2=0.34%, Correct=74.8					
	B	SE	Wald	df	Sig	Odds ratio
Most friends get drunk	1.181	0.129	83.267	1	0.000	3.257
Depression			9.365	2	0.009	
Somewhat depressed	0.182	0.156	1.369	1	0.242	1.200
Very depressed	0.475	0.158	9.010	1	0.003	1.607
Parental guidance			29.778	5	0.000	
Limits	0.881	0.195	20.383	1	0.000	2.414
Discourage use	0.170	0.230	0.546	1	0.460	1.185
Occasional mention	0.556	0.193	8.305	1	0.004	1.744
Thorough discussion	0.724	0.197	13.438	1	0.000	2.062
Favourable	0.817	0.227	12.893	1	0.000	2.263
Evening going out			49.652	2	0.000	
Sometimes	0.792	0.133	35.390	1	0.000	2.207
Almost daily	1.195	0.215	31.016	1	0.000	3.303
Hobbies less than weekly	0.463	0.133	12.193	1	0.000	1.589
Enjoyed the first drink	0.731	0.136	28.882	1	0.000	2.078
Got drunk first occasion	0.685	0.157	19.019	1	0.000	1.983
Age of first drink			29.920	6	0.000	
9 or less	1.431	0.297	23.279	1	0.000	4.183
10	0.975	0.306	10.151	1	0.001	2.652
11	1.018	0.292	12.180	1	0.000	2.768
12	0.895	0.273	10.739	1	0.001	2.448
13	0.700	0.271	6.670	1	0.010	2.014
14	0.539	0.279	3.742	1	0.053	1.715
Constant	−3.294	0.317	107.977	1	0.000	0.037
	Daily cigarette smoking					
	Cox and Snell R^2=0.26, Nagelkerke R^2=0.40%, Correct=83.7					
Female	0.781	0.174	20.167	1	0.000	2.183
Self-esteem			18.243	2	0.000	
Medium	0.397	0.206	3.732	1	0.053	1.487
Poor	0.849	0.203	17.564	1	0.000	2.338

(Continued)

Table 3.9 *(continued)* Logistic regression findings on binge drinking and daily cigarette smoking

	Daily cigarette smoking					
	Cox and Snell R^2=0.26, Nagelkerke R^2=0.40%, Correct=83.7					
Evening going out			18.863	2	0.000	
Sometimes	0.423	0.184	5.262	1	0.022	1.526
Almost daily	1.010	0.233	18.857	1	0.000	2.746
Most friends smoke	1.965	0.158	154.616	1	0.000	7.135
Hobbies less than weekly	0.524	0.157	11.146	1	0.001	1.689
Unsafe location first drink	0.445	0.161	7.665	1	0.006	1.560
Got drunk first occasion	0.441	0.168	6.861	1	0.009	1.554
Age of first drink			39.795	6	0.000	
9 or less	1.810	0.472	14.687	1	0.000	6.112
10	1.951	0.478	16.641	1	0.000	7.038
11	1.617	0.472	11.725	1	0.001	5.037
12	1.369	0.462	8.787	1	0.003	3.931
13	0.894	0.469	3.624	1	0.057	2.444
14	0.674	0.483	1.944	1	0.163	1.962
Constant	−5.133	0.496	107.199	1	0.000	0.006

df, degrees of freedom; SE, standard error; Sig, significance.

child's behaviour, are willing to discuss matters with their children, and listen to them in an open manner.

The experiences surrounding the first alcoholic drink may perhaps best be seen as giving some indication of this family ethos which, in turn, will play a part in determining the child's behaviour regarding substance use. Permissive parents with favourable attitudes to alcohol may allow their children to have a first real drink at an early age. A permissive atmosphere may encourage children to use alcohol, tobacco, and illicit drugs. This heavier use seems to occur despite the fact that, in permissive families favourable to alcohol (Table 3.9), the parents usually know about the first real drink and it is consumed in a safe environment. In families in which the parents discourage alcohol use, parents are less likely to know about the first real drink and it is less likely to take place in a safe environment, and, on average, the current substance use by these children at the age of 15 and 16 was low. However, for a minority in such families there would seem to be a degree of rebellion, with a less favourable result. This minority were likely to have their first real drink without their parent's knowledge and/or in a location outside the home. They can then go on to be heavier substance users at age 15 or 16. There are strong

Table 3.10 Logistic regression findings on cannabis use and use of other illicit drugs

	Lifetime cannabis use					
	Cox and Snell R^2=0.24, Nagelkerke R^2=0.34%, Correct=76.1					
	B	**SE**	**Wald**	**df**	**Sig**	**Odds ratio**
Internet almost daily	−0.370	0.143	6.654	1	0.010	0.691
Evening going out			32.619	2	0.000	
Sometimes	0.781	0.155	25.338	1	0.000	2.184
Almost daily	0.989	0.202	23.985	1	0.000	2.690
Friends use cannabis	2.188	0.217	101.806	1	0.000	8.916
Got drunk first occasion	0.730	0.149	24.079	1	0.000	2.074
Unsafe location first drink	0.485	0.138	12.325	1	0.000	1.625
Parents did not know first drink	0.305	0.151	4.078	1	0.043	1.356
Age of first drink			43.680	6	0.000	
9 or less	1.539	0.380	16.367	1	0.000	4.660
10	1.433	0.392	13.345	1	0.000	4.190
11	1.341	0.383	12.284	1	0.000	3.823
12	0.966	0.372	6.741	1	0.009	2.627
13	0.723	0.379	3.650	1	0.056	2.061
14	0.315	0.396	0.633	1	0.426	1.370
Constant	−4.414	0.415	112.913	1	0.000	0.012
	Lifetime use drugs other than cannabis					
	Cox and Snell R^2=0.16, Nagelkerke R^2=0.25%, Correct=79.5					
Depression			8.884	2	0.012	
Somewhat depressed	0.183	0.195	0.881	1	0.348	1.200
Very depressed	0.518	0.190	7.439	1	0.006	1.679
Evening going out			24.723	2	0.000	
Sometimes	0.706	0.171	17.145	1	0.000	2.027
Almost daily	0.970	0.210	21.248	1	0.000	2.638
Friends use cannabis	1.196	0.202	35.183	1	0.000	3.308
Got drunk first occasion	0.704	0.149	22.479	1	0.000	2.023
Age of first drink			65.557	6	0.000	
9 or less	1.698	0.410	17.154	1	0.000	5.463
10	1.540	0.421	13.400	1	0.000	4.665
11	1.069	0.419	6.520	1	0.011	2.912

(Continued)

Table 3.10 (*continued*) Logistic regression findings on cannabis use and use of other illicit drugs

	Lifetime use drugs other than cannabis					
	Cox and Snell R^2=0.16, Nagelkerke R^2=0.25%, Correct=79.5					
12	0.916	0.409	5.021	1	0.025	2.499
13	0.476	0.421	1.283	1	0.257	1.610
14	−0.161	0.460	0.123	1	0.726	0.851
Constant	−4.200	0.437	92.380	1	0.000	0.015

df, degrees of freedom; SE, standard error; Sig, significance.

parallels with clusters described by Baumrind (1991) in which parenting is considered in terms of commitment and the balance between being demanding and responsiveness. Authoritative parents who were both responsive and demanding were successful in protecting their adolescent children from substance use.

Of the 'early experience' variables the age of the first real drink bears the strongest relationships to current substance use. This relationship remains highly significant even after controlling for the current circumstances such as friend's drug use. The earlier the first real drink the more likely are binge drinking in the past 30 days, daily cigarette smoking, lifetime cannabis use, and lifetime use of other substances. Only a minority of students reported having become intoxicated on the first drinking occasion. This variable significantly predicts all four substance-use variables. Somewhat surprisingly there was no significant relationship between getting drunk on the first occasion and the age of that first experience with alcohol. However, if the student did get drunk on this first time, there was a strong tendency for the parents not to know about it. The other three 'early experience' variables—that is, enjoyment of the first real drink, its location, and parental knowledge that it took place—were highly significant predictors of substance use when considered singly. Even so, they were less likely to be predictors after controlling for other variables. Being able to remember the first ever sip of alcohol was not predictive of current substance use.

The variables measured here concerning the circumstances of the first 'real drink' seem particularly to tap the extent of permissiveness within the family towards alcohol and other drugs.

These findings are broadly consistent with several previous studies. The latter have indicated that early alcohol use is associated with later heavy and problematic drinking (Hingson and Kenkel 2004, York et al. 2004). Moreover, a study of young adults in the USA has shown that 'Children who are drinking by 7th grade are more likely to suffer employment problems, abuse other drugs, and commit criminal and violent acts once they reach adulthood' (RAND 2003). US evidence also shows that early 'alcohol abuse' was associated with elevated risk of problem drinking later in life (Substance Abuse and Mental Health Services Administration 2005). Dr Kenneth Moritsugu, the Acting Surgeon General of the USA, has issued the following strong statement:

> Research shows that young people who start drinking before the age of 15 are five times more likely to have alcohol-related problems later in life. New research also indicates that alcohol may harm the developing adolescent brain. The availability of this research provides more reasons than ever before for parents and other adults to protect the health and safety of our nation's children.

> (American Public Health Association 2007, p.1)

A Finnish study has also shown that early-onset drinking was associated with heavy drinking and alcohol-related problems among adult men. In addition, drinking before the age of 16 years was associated with adult heavy drinking among men and women (Pitkänen et al. 2005). In contrast, an analysis of 2003 UK ESPAD data indicated that early first drinking was a risk factor for teenage binge drinking only for certain groups of students (Afitska et al. 2008). It should also be noted that heavy drinking and alcohol-related problems among teenagers are generally low in countries where it has long been traditional for children to taste alcohol in a family context when they are young (Hibell et al. 2004). This suggests that culture pays an important role in influencing the possible links between early alcohol use and later behaviours. The present study supports the conclusion that the more permissive the family atmosphere the greater the likely substance use among UK teenagers. In spite of this, it should be noted that the large majority of these young people are unlikely to become chronic heavy users or drug dependents. It remains to be determined how the family ethos during childhood will play out when adolescents grow to adulthood.

What kind of country is the UK?

Recent trends in illicit drug use could usefully be considered in the light of evidence of other social trends in the UK. The latter may also be compared with other countries. A number of recent international comparisons do not show the UK in a favourable light. These include the following.

A report from the United Nations Childrens' Fund (UNICEF) (2007) revealed the findings of a study of the well-being of children in 21 industrialized countries. This examined 40 indicators of well-being, including health, poverty, and family relationships. The UK was ranked at the bottom of this league table, just below the USA, which was ranked number 20. The report noted that UK children were the unhappiest of those in all of the countries examined. UK children were also those most likely to use illicit drugs, were the heaviest drinkers, and were those most likely to have sex (Adamson 2007).

> Professor Jonathan Bradshaw from York University, one of the report's authors, put the UK's poor ratings down to long-term under-investment and a "dog-eat-dog" society.
>
> (BBC News Online, 14 February, 2007b)

The implications of this report were, predictably, controversial:

> The Conservatives accused the Chancellor, Gordon Brown, of failing a generation of children, although the report's author, Professor Jonathan Bradshaw of the University of York, said the result was a consequence of two decades of chronic underfunding in child health and education from 1979 to 1999....
>
> This report tells the truth about Brown's Britain," said George Osborne, the Shadow Chancellor. "After 10 years of his welfare and education policies, our children today have the lowest well-being in the developed world. The Chancellor has failed this generation of children and will fail the next if he's given a chance. We need a new approach."
>
> The Department of Education and Skills (Dfes) countered the report by saying that Unicef had used data that was several years old and did not reflect recent improvements in the welfare of British children, including the falling child poverty and teenage pregnancy rates.
>
> "Nobody can dispute that improving children's well-being is a real priority for this Government," said a spokeswoman.
>
> "There are now 700,000 fewer children living in relative poverty than in 1998–99, and we have halved the number of children living in absolute poverty," she said, adding that teenage pregnancy rates have fallen by 11 per cent since 1998 and were at their lowest levels for 20 years. But that did not stop a series of condemnations from academics and children's welfare groups, who highlighted dispiriting findings including the high proportion of 15-year-olds who aspire only to low-skilled work (35.3 per cent) and relatively small number of children who describe their peers as "kind and helpful": just 43.3 per cent.
>
> "We are not the poorest country in this league table, we are, in fact, the fifth richest," said Professor Bradshaw. "And yet we consistently come a long way behind the average... It's a pretty bleak picture."
>
> The lack of correlation between the UK's overall wealth and the prospects for its children prompted the Children's Commissioner, Professor Sir Albert Aynsley-Green, to say that society should look for the underlying causes of unhappiness and insecurity in the young.
>
> "There is a crisis at the heart of our society and we must not continue to ignore the impact of our attitudes towards children and young people and the effect that this has on their well-being," he said.
>
> (Times Online, 14 February, 2007)

Another report (also by Bradshaw) concluded that the UK was one of the worst countries in the Europe for young people to grow up in. The UK ranked 24th out of 29, ahead of only Bulgaria, Latvia, Lithuania, Malta, and Romania.

This report rated countries in relation to health, subjective well-being, personal relationships, material resources, education, behaviour and risks, housing, and the environment (Bradshaw and Richardson 2009).

A report funded by the prestigious charity, the Joseph Rowntree Foundation, examined trends in social inequality in Britain between 1968 and 2005. This concluded that social inequalities were growing, not declining. Moreover, the authors concluded that social inequality was as great as it had been forty years previously:

> Since 1970, area poverty and wealth in Britain have changed in significant ways. Over the past 15 years, more households have become poor, but fewer are very poor. Areas already wealthy have tended to become disproportionately wealthier, and we are seeing some evidence of increasing polarisation. In particular there are now areas in some of our cities where over half of all households are breadline poor.

> (Dorling et al. 2007, p.xiv; see also Joseph Rowntree Foundation 2007)

The fact that social inequalities were growing has recently been endorsed by the Government's National Equality Panel. This panel concluded that:

> there were profound and startling differences between deprived and affluent areas. Median total wealth in the poorest tenth of areas is only 6 per cent of the national figure, hourly wages are 40 per cent lower than in the most affluent areas, and only 55 per cent of working age adults in the poorest areas of England are employed.

> (Lloyd 2010)

In fact the UK is one of the most unequal of the developed countries. A review by the United Nations Development Program (2006) (cited by Wilkinson and Pickett 2009, p.7) revealed that the UK, together with the USA, Portugal, and Singapore, was ranked extremely poorly, with social inequality at twice the levels evident in Scandinavia and Japan. The Government's National Equality Panel (2010) reported that income inequalities in the UK were even greater than they had been 40 years earlier.

The UK ranks below several other countries on the United Nations Women's Empowerment Scale. It is ranked behind Sweden, Norway, Iceland, Denmark, Finland, New Zealand, and Canada (United Nations Development Program 2006). A similar picture of the position of UK women in relation to social, political, and economic empowerment has been reported by the World Economic Forum (Lopez-Claros and Zahidi 2005).

The UK has, by the standards of developed countries, high levels of income inequality. As noted by Wilkinson (2001) and Wilkinson and Pickett (2009) social inequality is associated with greater social and health problems. This is relevant for many forms of behaviour, including the heavy dependent use of illicit drugs. The latter frequently occur in the context of poverty and multiple problems such as unemployment, poor housing, and high crime rates (Dorn and South 1998, Lupton et al. 2002, Room 2005, Shaw et al. 2007). A recent report by the Organisation for Economic Co-operation and Development (OECD) noted that a high proportion of young people in the UK were not in school, training, or employment. Even so, UK children were rated as being materially well off and enjoyed a high quality of life (Organisation for Economic Co-operation and Development 2009). Marmot (2010) has noted the persistent substantial difference in mortality in the poorest neighbourhoods compared with the richest. The latter have life expectancies of 7 years better than the poorest. He has commented that priority objectives should be the following:

> Reduce inequalities in the early development of physical and emotional health, and cognitive, linguistic, and social skills.
> Ensure high quality maternity services, parenting programmes, childcare and early years education to meet need across the social gradient.
> Build the resilience and well-being of young children across the social gradient.

> (Marmot 2010, p.22)

The consequences associated with illicit drug use are considered in the following chapter. It is important to emphasize that, as in the case of the legal drugs (alcohol and tobacco) illicit drug use is subject to changing social fashions and norms. Most people who use illicit drugs in the UK do not become chronic heavy users or drug-dependent. Moreover, many of those who experiment with illicit drugs when they are young either give up drug use completely or remain only occasional, light users.

Chapter 4

The consequences of drug use: the good, the bad, and the ugly

The United Kingdom has the highest level of dependent drug use and among the highest levels of recreational drug use in Europe.
(Reuter and Stevens 2007, p.7)

More than 100 police officers swept through 23 addresses in London today, and smashed what Scotland Yard described as the largest cocaine and money laundering ring ever uncovered in the UK. Police arrested 10 men and two women in connection with the Colombia-based drugs cartel. Searches were ongoing at a number of homes and businesses in east London, Holloway in north London and Brixton in south London. Most of those held in London were foreign nationals from South America. The arrests formed the final phase of a two-year international operation targeting a highly organised cocaine importation and money laundering ring, Scotland Yard said. Detective Chief Superintendent Sharon Kerr said the investigation was the first time in the history of policing that Scotland Yard had been able to take out an entire network of individuals from top organisers to people selling drugs on the street. The cartel had netted in excess of £100m in the last six months, Det Ch Supt Kerr said.
(Left 2003)

The Dutch want to ban the sale of magic mushrooms. Amsterdam's emergency services had 55 call-outs to

mushroom-related incidents in 2004 and 128 in 2006.
Most involved young Britons.
(Observer, 27 April, 2008, p.38)

In 2006 and 2007 a new method of smuggling
emerged, surface skimming, semi submersible, home
made submarines were captured from Thailand to
Spain to Colombia. In 2008 the number spotted had
already reached the 2007 count. These craft often had
sophisticated electronics for evading capture. To get
some idea of the logistical scale of these things, a 100ft
long Russian designed submarine was captured in
Colombia's capital Bogata, 7,500 ft above sea level.
(Oobject 2008)

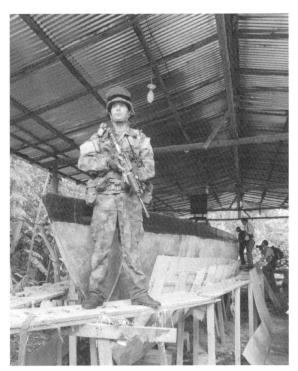

Colombian marines secure an illegal shipyard where a midget submersible was under
construction in Playa del Vigia, June 2009

Credit: Getty Images.

During February 2009 the International Narcotics
Control Board noted that Internet dealing in both
illicit and unauthorised prescription drugs had risen
to "alarming levels"
(Campbell 2009a)

This chapter reviews recent evidence on the extent and patterns of both
the positive effects (such as enjoyment and allied social and psychological
benefits) and the negative effects of illicit drug use among people in the UK.
Negative effects include drug-related crimes, accidents, overdoses, injuries,
illness (e.g. hepatitis C, HIV/AIDS, drug dependence, and psychiatric illness),
and premature mortality. The latter particularly involves young people. This
chapter also presents new evidence from the 2007 European School Survey
Project on Alcohol and other Drugs (ESPAD 2007; noted above) related to the
consequences of drug use among UK teenagers.

Positive aspects and motivation to take drugs

Samuel Taylor Coleridge declared that sniffing nitrous oxide was the 'most
unmingled pleasure' that he ever enjoyed. Most people use mind-altering
drugs, be they legal, prescribed, or illicit, for positive reasons. Studies routinely
show that most initial use of recreational drugs such as alcohol, cannabis,
cocaine, ecstasy, or tobacco is motivated by a mixture of curiosity and the
wish to fit in socially with friends and acquaintances. Thereafter, if drug use
continues, enjoyment of drug effects and the reinforcement this provides is a
major motivating factor. People enjoy taking drugs. In the case of prescribed
drugs, use is generally motivated by the belief or hope that they will improve
the quality of life, for example by allaying anxieties or depressed mood. Millions
of people use illicit or controlled drugs at least a few times in their lives. It is
obvious that most of this use is motivated by positive factors and that
enormous numbers of people really enjoy drug effects, just as they enjoy
the effects of the most popular recreational drugs, alcohol and tobacco.
Individuals who use drugs many times or for extended periods frequently
attribute a number of subjective or perceived positive consequences to drug
use. It is commonplace for recreational users to declare that taking a drug
enhances their ability to appreciate music, food, scenery, sex, or life in general.
Some people report that drug use enables them to attain or relish spiritual
experiences or transcendental states. Many people clearly enjoy drug-induced
'disinhibition', reporting that this enables them to relax and feel more confident and sociable. Moreover, social drug use provides companionship and

personal support. Membership of a drug-using group may also confer social status and excitement (Goode 1970. 1972, Plant 1975). Ecstasy users have reported that using this drug produces a positive mood, with feelings of intimacy and closeness to others. Other reported effects included insight, combined with 'perceptual and sensual enlightenment' (Solowij et al. 2006). The subjectively positive effects of drug use may have negative results, at least for some people. Parrott et al. (2001), examining self-reported drug effects among young people in London, Manchester, Padua, and Rome concluded that:

> The current findings show that as an individual moves up the drug-usage scale, self-reported positive moods and experiences remain unchanged, while psychiatric symptoms and psychobiological problems increase.

> (Parrott et al. 2001, p.81)

Crowley et al. (1998) have pointed out that cannabis use is a reinforcing activity. They further concluded that:

> for adolescents with conduct problems cannabis use is not benign, and that the drug potently reinforces cannabis-taking, producing both dependence and withdrawal.

> (Crowley et al. 1998, p.27)

A similar view has been expressed by O'Brien et al. (1998). The latter have stated that that abundant clinical evidence supports the view that:

> compulsion to resume drug taking is an important part of the addiction syndrome.

> (O'Brien et al. 1998, p.15)

Comeau et al. (2001) concluded from a study of US adolescents that:

> Across alcohol, cigarettes, and marijuana, coping, enhancement, and conformity motives appear relatively "risky" in that they have been closely related to heavy and/or problem use...Cooper, M.L., 1994. Motivations for alcohol use among adolescents: development and validation of a four-factor model. Patterns suggest that those who use substances to change internal states (i.e., for coping and enhancement reasons) may use more heavily and/or chronically than others.... Additionally, it appears that using substances for negative reinforcement reasons (i.e., coping and conformity) may represent a relatively maladaptive style of use that results in problems.... In contrast, social motives appear to be associated with a relatively lighter, less problematic style of substance use and thus are considered less risky reasons for use.

> (Comeau et al. 2001, p.803)

The topic of illicit drugs causes enormous concern. One of the reasons for this is the fear that 'drugs' have a particular appeal to inexperienced, vulnerable young people. It has been suggested that illicit drug use should be included as one of 18 social indicators by which schools in England and Wales are assessed (Lipsett 2008). It is important to bear in mind that the consequences of drug use depend upon several factors. These include the prevalence of use as well as the chemistry of the substance. It should be emphasized that the health damage caused by the most widely used (and legal) drugs alcohol and tobacco is much more widespread than that associated with illicit drugs. Even so, there is good reason for regarding the adverse consequences of illicit drug use as a serious problem. The respective scale of alcohol, tobacco, and illicit drug problems is considered below. Fortunately, as outlined in the previous chapter, most of those who experiment with illicit drugs do so in moderation. They do not become either heavy or chronic users.

It has to be emphasized that the production, distribution, and sale of illicit drugs (as well as of alcohol, tobacco, and prescription drugs) are global activities. As elaborated eloquently by Alexander (2008) the demand for these substances is massive and international.

Mortality and morbidity

It should be acknowledged that, while the problems associated with illicit drugs are considerable, they are in many ways dwarfed by those associated with the popular and widely used legal substances, beverage alcohol and tobacco. The World Health Organization has described the scale of drug-related health problems in the following terms:

There are a number of disorders resulting from the use of psychoactive substances including alcohol, opioids such as opium or heroin, cannabinoids such as marijuana, sedatives and hypnotics, cocaine, other stimulants, hallucinogens, tobacco and volatile solvents. These conditions include acute intoxication, harmful use, dependence and psychotic disorders. Tobacco and alcohol are the substances which are used most widely across the globe and which pose the most serious public health consequences.

Prevalence: Today, one in three adults or 1.2 billion people use tobacco worldwide. By 2025, the number is expected to rise to more than 1.6 billion. Tobacco was estimated to account for 4 million annual deaths by 1998. This is expected to rise to 8.4 million deaths by 2020. In the African region, tobacco consumption is estimated to be on the increase, more than in any other region of the world.

Worldwide, there are an estimated 70 million people who have alcohol use disorders, including harmful use and dependence - 78% of whom remain untreated. The rate of alcohol use disorder for men is 2.8% and for women 0.5%. An estimated 5 million people worldwide inject illicit drugs - there is a high prevalence of HIV infection among injecting drug users, making it a major public health concern.

(World Health Organization 2002)

Seventeen people a week are now being admitted to accident and emergency departments after taking cocaine.

(BBC News Online, 13 July, 2009b)

The European Monitoring Centre for Drugs and Alcohol Addiction (EMCDDA 2008) has reported that:

> In 2005–06, drug-induced deaths accounted for 3.5% of all deaths of Europeans 15–39 years old, with opioids being found in around 70% of them.
>
> (EMCDDA 2008, p.13)

The United Nations Office on Drugs and Crime (2005) has reported that the vast scale of illicit drug use is accompanied by a correspondingly huge level of adverse effects. These include damage to the individual's health and to society: problems include blood-borne diseases, premature deaths, mental health problems, social disruption, crime, and a host of other consequences such as economic disruption, political instability, terrorism, and corruption. In some countries drug dealers have the resources to evade due legal processes and to undermine democratic institutions.

As already noted, 100 000 UK deaths each year are associated with tobacco smoking and over 8000 are associated with alcohol (Royal College of Physicians 2001b, British Medical Association 2008). Tobacco smoking was associated with an incredible 6 300 000 deaths in the UK during the second half of the twentieth century. Illicit drugs are connected to fewer than 3000 deaths annually (DrugScope 2008).

The calculation of the number of people in the UK who die because of their drug use is not straightforward, as noted by DrugScope:

> There is no one organization that collects information about drug-related deaths, for all of the UK.
> There is no one definition of what we mean by drug-related deaths. For example, it could include:
> - people who are dependent on drugs and overdose
> - suicides by overdose of people who have no previous history of using drugs
> - accidental poisoning or overdose
> - ecstasy related deaths where people have died from overheating through dancing non-stop in hot clubs rather than from the direct effect of the drugs
> - deaths associated with cigarette smoking
> - deaths from accidents where people are drunk or under the influence of drugs
> - murders and manslaughters where people are drunk or under the influence of drugs
> - deaths from driving while drunk or intoxicated
> - deaths from AIDS and other blood borne viruses such as hepatitis C among injecting drug users
> - deaths which had nothing to do with the presence of a drug in the body. Cause of death is recorded on death certificates but doctors may not mention drugs, even where drugs might be involved. Despite these difficulties there are estimates of the possible number of deaths associated with different drugs.
>
> (DrugScope 2008)

A study was conducted that examined every person in the UK known to be addicted to heroin in 1954 and all further cases of this addiction notified from then until the end of 1964 (Bewley 1965). Fifty-seven heroin addicts were known in 1954 and 450 new cases were added in the following 10 years. Research covered the 507 recorded heroin addicts between 1954 and 1964. The rate of appearance of new cases has steadily increased. Over 80% of all addicts remained addicted or died. Present methods of dealing with this addiction are ineffectual. Preventive measures are recommended, including limitations on prescribing heroin for addicts (see Chapter 9).

The Office for National Statistics provides a record of the number of people in England and Wales who have died from drug overdoses:

> The number of deaths related to drug poisoning in England and Wales increased each year from 1993 to a peak in 1999, and then began to decline. After increases in 2001 and 2004, the number fell to 2,570 deaths in 2006. This was a decrease of 7 per cent compared with 2005 and the lowest recorded number since 1995.
>
> This trend mainly reflects changes in the mortality for drug poisoning among males who made up over two thirds of these deaths in 2006. The gap between the number of male and female deaths has increased since 1993. From the late 1990s there have been twice as many deaths in males than females.
>
> The number of female deaths fell by 10 per cent between 2005 and 2006, to 783 deaths, after no discernable trend over the last 13 years. This was the lowest number since records began in 1993, when there were 865 deaths.
>
> The underlying cause of these deaths reflects the verdict of the coroner and varies by sex. Among males broadly similar numbers of deaths were due to drug abuse/ dependence (30 per cent), accidental poisoning (30 per cent) and intentional self-poisoning/poisoning of undetermined intent (39 per cent). The majority of deaths among females were intentional selfpoisonings/poisonings of undetermined intent (64 per cent of deaths related to drug poisoning in 1993-2006 combined).
>
> There were 713 deaths involving heroin or morphine in 2006. This was the lowest recorded number since 1999 and a fall of 15 per cent from 2005. The number of deaths involving methadone however increased by 10 per cent between 2005 and 2006 when there were 241. This was not as high as the peak of 437 in 1997.
>
> Deaths involving cocaine continued to increase in 2006 to 190 deaths. This was the highest number of deaths where cocaine was mentioned since records began in 1993, when 11 deaths mentioned cocaine. The number mentioning amphetamines fell by 11 per cent between 2005 and 2006, to 92 deaths, but over half of these were accounted for by deaths mentioning ecstasy.

(Office for National Statistics 2008a)

Williams et al. (2005) have reported that during 2002–3 there were 7380 hospital admissions in England and Wales for 'mental and behavioural disorders due to controlled drugs'. The corresponding number related to alcohol was 18863. Patton et al. (2009) have reported that the most common cause of mortality among those aged 10–24 years in the UK is road traffic accident. Russell Viner, one of the authors of the Patton et al. report, has noted that many of these accidents are associated with alcohol and illicit drug use (Boseley 2009).

As previously noted, Shaw et al. (2009) have produced a weighty and invaluable overview of detailed statistical information related to illicit drug use and drug-related problems in the nine regions of England. They cite evidence related to 46 indicators of individual, community, and populations 'implications' of drug use. The authors concluded that:

> The prevalence of opiate and or crack cocaine use, the rate of individuals in contact with structured drug treatment and the number of drug related hospital admissions were all higher in more deprived regions of England in comparison to more affluent regions.
>
> (Shaw al. 2009, p.18)

The overall regional rates of individuals in contact with structured drug treatment services are shown in Table 4.1. As this table shows, the rates of contact with structured drug-treatment services were especially high in north-west England, followed by London, Yorkshire and Humberside, and north-east England. The regional rates of drug-related deaths in England are shown in Table 4.2. The highest drug-related mortally rates were evident in north-east England. They were also relatively high in north-west and south-west England and Yorkshire and Humberside. In fact rates of drug-related mortality in England have declined. Between 2001 and 2007 they fell from 4.95 people per 100 000 population to 4.2 people per 100 000. The number of such deaths in 2007 was recorded as being 1479.

Table 4.1 Rates per 1000 of population of people aged 15–64 in contact with structured drug-treatment services in England

Region	Males	Females	Total
North east	9.81	3.44	6.59
North west	11.48	4.57	7.99
Yorkshire and Humberside	11.20	4.42	7.80
East Midlands	7.47	2.78	5.13
West Midlands	8.40	2.96	5.68
Eastern England	5.20	2.26	3.73
London	9.27	3.76	7.96
South east	4.89	1.99	3.44
South west	8.39	3.35	5.86
England	8.33	3.27	5.78

(*Source*: Shaw et al. 2009, p.149; figures from National Drug Treatment Monitoring System (NDTMS).)

Table 4.2 Rates per 1 000 000 of population of people aged 15–64 dying from 'drug misuse' in England (2007)

Region	Males	Females	Total
North east	8.50	1.87	5.17
North west	7.69	2.20	4.94
Yorkshire and Humberside	7.75	1.58	4.68
East Midlands	5.73	1.37	3.56
West Midlands	7.44	1.25	4.35
Eastern England	5.31	1.08	3.19
London	6.47	1.02	3.75
South east	6.36	1.61	3.98
South west	8.00	1.61	4.81
England	6.91	1.49	4.20

(*Source*: Shaw et al 2009, p.173; figures from the Office for National Statistics.)

The number of drug-related deaths in Scotland has been fluctuating, but has risen sharply in recent years. The popular press have reported this in terms of the death of the '*Trainspotting* generation'. It would probably be more appropriate to call these the Thatcher generation. In fact deaths have increased among drug users of all ages. The number of drug-related deaths rose by just over 50% between 2002 and 2008. This is shown in Table 4.3.

Recent trends in Scottish drug-related deaths have been summarized thus:

> On the basis of the definition used for these statistics, there were 574 drug-related deaths in 2008, 119 (26 per cent) more than in 2007 and 325 (131 per cent) more than in 1998. The number of drug-related deaths has risen in eight of the past ten years: the long-term trend appears to be steadily upwards.
>
> Males accounted for 80 per cent of the drug-related deaths in 2008.
>
> In 2008, there were 211 drug-related deaths of people aged 25-34 (representing 37 per cent of all drug-related deaths) and 174 drug-related deaths of 35-44 year olds (30 per cent). In addition, 92 people aged under 25 died (16 per cent), as did 97 people aged 45 and over (17 per cent).
>
> The Health Board areas which accounted for the majority of the 574 drug-related deaths in 2008 were:
>
> Greater Glasgow & Clyde - 197 (34 per cent); Lothian - 94 (16 per cent); and Tayside - 53 (9 per cent).
>
> (General Register Office for Scotland 2009, p.3)

Worldwide blood-borne viruses spread by injecting drug use account for a considerable mortality both by direct infection and from subsequent sexual spread. Some consider that injecting drug use and the reuse of contaminated

Table 4.3 Drug-related deaths in Scotland (2002–8)

	Number of drug-related deaths					
Year	2002	2003	2004	2005	2006	2008
Scotland (total)	382	317	356	336	421	574
Ayrshire and Arran	33	19	20	15	25	40
Borders	–	2	2	7	2	7
Dumfries and Galloway	9	9	7	7	5	9
Fife	12	12	17	21	19	37
Forth Valley	24	12	16	14	24	23
Grampian	47	37	39	23	47	41
Gt Glasgow and Clyde (1)	152	131	151	111	162	197
Highland (1)	13	10	12	13	12	24
Lanarkshire	37	25	33	40	40	44
Lothian	39	40	36	57	46	94
Orkney	–	–	–	–	1	1
Shetland	1	–	–	1	2	1
Tayside	14	19	23	26	35	53
Western Isles	1	1	–	1	1	3
Argyll and Clyde	31	27	35	29	36	No data
Gt Glasgow and Clyde pt	26	24	31	26	35	No data
Highland pt	5	3	4	3	1	No data
Gt Glasgow (2)	126	107	120	85	127	No data
Highland (2)	8	7	8	10	11	No data

(*Source*: General Register Office for Scotland 2008, 2009)

medical equipment has some part to play in the rapid transmission of HIV in sub-Saharan Africa. In Asia at present there is evidence of epidemic HIV transmission among the growing drug-injecting populations.

Injecting drug use is now seen as a worldwide cause of HIV infection and transmission. An estimated 15.9 million people inject drugs the largest numbers of injectors have been found in China, the USA, and Russia, where mid-estimates of HIV prevalence among injectors were 12%, 16%, and 37%, respectively (Mathers et al. 2008). HIV prevalence in Kenya has in one study been found to be 68%–88% in injecting drug users, and the figure is 28% in South Africa. In Russia methadone and alternatives are banned and these treatments and provision of needle-exchange facilities are largely unavailable in most of Africa (Csete et al. 2009)

Development of drug dependence

It is certain that some, probably many, of those who are dependent upon illicit drugs at some time in their lives are not recorded by official agencies. An indication of the widespread nature of drug dependence has been provided by a recent survey conducted by DrugScope (2009b). This revealed that 19% of UK adults had at some time in their lives either been drug dependent or had witnessed such dependence in somebody close to them, such as a relative or friend. This experience was reportedly particularly high among those aged 18–34 years, involving 27% of this group. One person in 50 reported having been drug-dependent at some time.

> DrugScope commissioned the poll to find out more about public attitudes to drug users and drug treatment. The findings suggest that the public's views are more sympathetic than may sometimes be assumed by policymakers and commentators. The majority - 80 per cent - of those surveyed agreed that "people can become addicted to drugs because of other problems in their lives" whereas only 35 per cent agreed with the statement "there is no excuse for drug addiction – it is always the individual's fault." Overwhelming support for drug treatment was revealed, with 88 per cent of respondents agreeing that "people who have become addicted to drugs need help and support to get their lives back on track" and 77 per cent agreeing that investment in drug treatment is "a sensible use of government money…"
>
> The sympathetic response of the majority of people surveyed is in sharp contrast to much media reporting and public discourse around drug users. People with a drug dependency are among the most marginalised groups in society, and stigma and discrimination are real barriers to recovery for many; a recent poll found that two thirds of employers would not employ someone with a history of heroin or crack use, even if they were otherwise suitable for the job.
>
> (DrugScope 2009b, p.1)

Treatment costs

It appears that the treatment of drug users is, by at least one measure, superior to that for people who have alcohol-related problems. The House of Commons Public Administration Committee (2009) has reported that National Health Service expenditure on people undergoing treatment for drug problems was £1744, while that for people with alcohol-related problems was only £197 (Campbell 2009b).

Road traffic accidents

Illicit drugs are certainly implicated with road traffic accidents, but there appear to be no reliable figures on the scale of this. The UK Department of Transport has noted that 10% of young male drivers have reported drug driving. As noted in Chapter 3, there is currently no approved equivalent to the alcohol breathalyser for use in detecting drug use. A £2.3 million media campaign launched in August 2009 bizarrely highlighted the fact that the police might detect supposed evidence of drug use by observing dilated or constricted pupils. It is doubtful that such observations would have much credibility in court. This approach is reminiscent of attempting to detect alcohol-impaired driving by asking a person to walk along a chalk line on the floor. The Department of Transport emphasized the adverse effects on a driver's abilities of cannabis, cocaine, amphetamines, and ecstasy (BBC News Online, 17 August, 2009c).

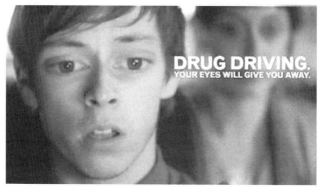

Credit: Department of Transport.

Benzodiazepine dependence

Benzodiazepines were originally made available during the 1950s. They were viewed as a safer alternative to barbiturates. It transpired that patients who received prescriptions for these drugs developed tolerance and dependence (Petursson and Lader 1981, Owen and Tyrer 1983, Lader and Higgit 1986, Ashton 1994). Use of these drugs was high during the early 1980s when up to a remarkable 11% of the population were believed to be taking these drugs. This level had dropped to around 3% by 1986. Benzodiazepines remain a cause for concern. Sir Liam Donaldson, the UK Government's Chief Medical Advisor, issued a warning about these drugs in 2004. This reminded doctors that benzodiazepines should not be used for treating mild anxiety. Moreover, these drugs should only be used for short-term treatment (Department of Health 2004).

The European School Survey Project on Alcohol and other Drugs (ESPAD) has been noted in the previous chapter. This study relates to 15- and 16-year-old school students in Europe. ESPAD teenagers were asked whether or not they had experienced any problems due to their own use of drugs. The results of

Table 4.4 Experience of individual problems related to personal drug use in past year

Type of problem	Boys (%)	Girls (%)
Accident or injury	5	4
Performed poorly at work or school	5	4
Hospitalised or admitted to accident and emergency department	1	1
Serious problem with friends	3	3
Serious problem with parents	4	3

(*Source*: Hibell et al. 2009, p.351)

this are shown in Table 4.4. Only a small number of teenagers reported having experienced such problems. It should be noted that far more teenagers reported adverse effects associated with drinking alcohol. Levels of alcohol-related problems experienced by UK teenagers included accidents and injuries (26%), poor performance at school or work (12%), being hospitalized or admitted to an accident and emergency department (3%), having relationship problems with friends (17%) or parents (18%), regretting having had sexual intercourse (11%) or unprotected sex (11%), and delinquency problems such as fighting (17%), being victimized by robbery or theft (4%), and getting into trouble with police (15%).

ESPAD teenagers were asked to indicate what forms of legal or illicit drug use they assessed as involving 'great risk'. Among UK respondents the highest proportions who responded in this way related to regular ecstasy use (75%), regular amphetamine use (68%), regular cannabis smoking (61%), smoking one or more packs of cigarettes each day (59%), and consuming four or five drinks each day (58%).

Information from the 2007 ESPAD survey was used for a number of specialized analyses. These included an examination of cannabis-related problems and a 'psychosocial module'. Both of these sub-studies used data from the UK part of ESPAD. They are now briefly considered. The examination of cannabis-related problems was conducted by Piontek et al. (2008a). These authors examined school students in 17 ESPAD countries in relation to their responses to an instrument known as the Cannabis Abuse Screening Test (CAST) (Beck and Legleye 2003). The latter consists of the following six questions:

1 Have you ever smoked cannabis before midday?

2 Have you ever smoked cannabis when you were alone?

3 Have you ever had memory problems when you smoke cannabis?

4 Have friends or family members ever told you outright that you ought to reduce your cannabis use?

5 Have you ever tried to reduce or stop your cannabis use?

6 Have you ever had problems because of your use of cannabis (arguments, fights, accidents, bad results at school, etc.)?

Analysis of responses to CAST were examined in relation to 7297 teenagers who had used cannabis in the past year. UK teenagers had medium-low rankings on the first five CAST items, but ranked highest in relation to number 6 (arguments, fights, accidents, bad results at school). In spite of this the overall proportion of 'high-risk' cannabis users in the UK was ranked below that in Cyprus, Greece, the Isle of Man, Italy, and Monaco. It was concluded that '…at population level the prevalence of high-risk users increases with the prevalence of cannabis use' (Beck and Legleye 2003, p.169)

An examination of psychosocial factors among adolescents in ESPAD countries was carried out by Kokkevi and Fotiou (2009). This work was prompted by the fact that it is well established that psychopathology is associated with heavy drug use (Johnston et al. 1996, Glantz and Leshner, 2000). Twenty ESPAD national research teams included at least some of a number of items that constituted the ESPAD psychosocial module. These related to self-esteem, depression, anomie, antisocial behaviour, items on running away from home, and thoughts of self-harm and attempted suicide. The countries that elicited information about these topics were Armenia, Austria, Belgium (Flemish part), Bulgaria, Croatia, Cyprus, the Faroe Islands, Finland, Germany, Greece, Hungary, Iceland, Ireland, the Isle of Man, Latvia, Romania, Slovakia, Slovenia, the UK, and Ukraine. A total of 57 858 teenagers answered at least one of the psychosocial module items. The analysis showed that:

> There is a graded association between intensity of smoking (number of cigarettes per day) and the percentage of students exceeding the cut-off points for the scales of depressive mood, low self-esteem, antisocial behaviour and anomie. The same pattern is observed for the frequency of alcohol use in the last month…, for drunkenness in the lat 12 months, for cannabis use in the last 12 months…. And for the lifetime use of any legal drug except cannabis… A strong association is observed between the number of psychosocial risk factors (from 0 to 4 or more) and the intensity of frequency of the substance use variables.

> (Kokkevi and Fotiou 2009, pp.178–80)

Currie et al. (2008), considering findings from the 2005/6 Health Behaviour of School Children (HBSC) study, have concluded:

> Although cannabis use may be normative, and there is evidence to suggest that young people who use cannabis in modest doses are better adjusted and have better social skills than non-users or heavyusers, frequent use of cannabis is associated with negative outcomes. Population studies among cannabis users have identified increased rates of externalizing disorders such as juvenile offending and conduct problems, and,

to a lesser extent, internalizing problems such as psychosis and depression. These problems may both predate and be exacerbated by cannabis. Along with other substance use (such as tobacco and alcohol), cannabis use has been listed as among the risk factors for psychiatric morbidity.

(Currie et al. 2008, p.139)

Drug overdoses

The Office for National Statistics (2006) has reported that:

In 2004, the number of deaths involving heroin or morphine rose to 744 (from 591 in 2003), following a decline over the previous four years from the highest recorded number of 926 deaths in 2000.

These figures related to England and Wales.

Occupation

They tried to make me go to rehab, I said no, no, no
Yes I've been black but when I come back you'll know know know
I ain't got the time and if my daddy thinks I'm fine
He's tried to make me go to rehab, I won't go go go.

(Amy Winehouse 2006)

It is well established that heavy drinking and alcohol-related problems as well as tobacco smoking and its ill effects are especially widespread in some occupations rather than others. This has been attributed to factors such as occupational culture, peer pressure, availability in the workplace, travelling, unsocial hours, and stress (Plant 1979, Office for National Statistics 2007). It has long been obvious that many rock-and-roll musicians (e.g. the Beatles, the Rolling Stones, Pete Docherty, George Michael, Amy Winehouse, and many more) have used drugs and that some (e.g. Janis Joplin, Jim Morrison, Jimi Hendrix, Phil Lynott of Thin Lizzy, Keith Moon, Elvis Presley, and Michael Jackson) have allegedly died from drug-related causes. A study of musicians who had produced 'the all-time top 1000 albums from the music genres rock, punk, rap, R&B, electronica and new age' revealed high levels of early mortality linked with alcohol or illicit drugs (Bellis et al. 2007). The authors concluded that:

Pop stars can suffer high levels of stress in environments where alcohol and drugs are widely available, leading to health-damaging risk behaviour. However, their behaviour can also influence would-be stars and devoted fans.

(Bellis et al. 2007, p.896)

There is no doubt that some popular songs have included references to drugs. Many more have been alleged to do so because of obvious or ambiguous phrases such as 'everybody must get stoned', 'day tripper', 'I've got speed',

'E's are good', and many more. Drug use by pop stars, actors, and other famous people and the effect that this might have on their millions of admirers has been criticized by many people since the birth of popular music and other forms of entertainment. The latter has always been viewed as a subversive threat by some people. During 2008 Philip Emafo, President of the International Narcotics Control Board (INCB), criticized what he viewed as the lenient treatment accorded to celebrity drug users, a view officially endorsed by his organization (International Narcotics Control Board 2008a). In fairness, it should be noted that many films (such as *Trainspotting* and *Traffic*) and songs portrayed a more thoughtful and balanced, or distinctly anti-drug message. This too may be influential.

> I have made very big decision
> I'm goin to try to nullify my life
> cause when the blood begins to flow
> When it shoots up the droppers neck
> When I'm closing in on death.
>
> *(Lou Reed 1964)*

Drug-user careers

As previously noted, neither drug use nor drug dependence are necessarily permanent conditions. A dramatic illustration of this fact was provided by the experiences of large numbers of US veterans after the Vietnam War. Many of these individuals had begun to use heroin while in Vietnam, but ceased to use the drug after returning home (Robins 1973, 1974, 1975, Robins et al. 1974, 1975, 1980, Helzer et al. 1985). If, how, and when people begin, continue, or cease to use drugs depends upon a host of situational factors. Numerous examples of this have been described at times. These include the upsurge in the use of heroin in Crawley during the 1970s (Mott and Rathod 1976; note the impressive 33-year follow-up by Rathod et al. 2005) and drug use among socially excluded youth in the north of England during the 1990s and between 1999 and 2001 (Parker et al. 1998, MacDonald 2003).

The children of problem drug users

The possible impact on people of having one or both parents who are heavy or problematic drug users has been mentioned in Chapter 3. This subject has been addressed in detail by the Advisory Council on the Misuse of Drugs (2003, 2007). The 2003 report concluded that:

- ◆ There are between 250,000 and 350,000 children of problem drug users in the UK: about 1 child for every problem drug user.

♦ Parental problem drug use causes serious harm to children at every age from conception to adulthood.

♦ Reducing the harm to children from parental problem drug use should become a main objective of policy and practice.

♦ Effective treatment of the parent can have major benefits for the child.

♦ By working together, services can take many practical steps to protect and improve the health and well-being of affected children.

♦ The number of affected children is only likely decrease when the number of problem drug users decreases.

(Advisory Council on the Misuse of Drugs 2003)

In fact, although the children of problem drug users are obviously an 'at-risk' group, caution is needed when reaching conclusions about them. As noted by Velleman and Templeton (2003) it should not be assumed that all drug users are hopeless parents (though some are) or that all such children will necessarily be severely harmed.

The adulteration of drugs

The risks that illicit drugs might be dangerously contaminated or adulterated have sometimes been deliberately exaggerated as a means, it is hoped, of discouraging people from using them. In fact some research suggests that such adulteration is unusual (Coomber 1997a, 1997b, 1997c, 1997d, 1999). In spite of this drug supplies are sometimes unsafe. This is elaborated elsewhere. It has been reported that some supplies of cocaine in England were being adulterated. The proportion of supply that was pure had fallen from 63% in 1984 to only 26% at the end of 2007. It was noted that such adulteration was normally by mixing cocaine with painkillers and sugars (Travis 2009a, p.9).

Clearly drug-related harm accumulates as time goes on and unfolding problems of HIV/AIDS in Asian countries and anthrax epidemics in the UK are further examples which will emerge over the next few years. The aging population of drug users is already showing the longer-term damage and consequences of past and continued drug taking and new horrors are likely to become evident as the hepatitis C epidemic matures. The incubation period of hepatitis C is two or more decades so the long-term caseload has only just begun to present to clinical specialists. The consequences of excessive drug use and the associated alcohol and tobacco indulgence are likely to add to the premature illness and deaths in drug takers.

Chapter 5

Drug-control policies: a question of balance

There are naysayers who believe a global fight against illegal drugs is unwinnable. I say emphatically they are wrong. Our slogan for the Special Session is "A Drug Free World - We Can Do It!" The United Nations and the International Drug Control Programme (UNDCP) will help lead the way. – Towards a drug-free world by 2008 - we can do it.
(Pino Arlacchi, United Nations Under-Secretary-General 1998)

If the government can't keep drugs away from inmates who are locked in steel cages, surrounded by barbed wire, watched by armed guards, drug-tested, strip-searched, X-rayed, and videotaped–how can it possibly stop the flow of drugs to an entire nation?
(Ron Crickenberger)

The main options: prohibition, harm minimization, or legalization?

In the twentieth century, political leaders and governments throughout the world supported drug prohibition and constructed a global drug prohibition system. They did so because of the influence of the USA and its allies at the [United Nations]. … they also did so because drug prohibition, drug demonisation and anti-drug campaigns were very useful/especially to politicians, the police, the military, and the media.

(Levine 2003, p.145)

There are many different views on the best way to reduce drug-related problems. Drugs are controversial. Opinions on the best way to deal with them cover the entire spectrum from legalization to tight controls backed up by severe penalties. In fact most of the 'official' and public debate about drug policy reflects the view that drugs are intrinsically 'bad' and should somehow be controlled. The authors of this book do not wish to embrace any particular approach to drug control. They do not believe that any single known approach is a magic solution, offering a panacea to something as complex and multi-faceted as drug use and its associated adverse effects. Even so, it is hoped that this chapter will provide an insight into some of the debates and arguments that relate to the nature and status of drug use and the options that are available with which to respond to it. It might also be possible to envisage ways of mitigating the damaging consequences outlined in the previous chapter without having to embark on a political crusade or to turn around the juggernaut of international condemnation of drug use and drug users.

Prohibition

To a man with a hammer, everything looks like a nail.

(Mark Twain)

The first meeting to consider international drug problems took place in Shanghai in 1909. This paved the way for the first international drug-control treaty, the International Opium Convention. This was signed in The Hague in 1912. This treaty sought to achieve the following:

the gradual suppression of the abuse of opium, morphine, and cocaine and also of the drugs prepared or derived from these substances, which give rise or might give rise to similar abuses.

International drug controls were subsequently extended, and were unified by the Single Convention on Narcotic Drugs in 1961. This has been described in the following words:

The Single Convention codified all existing multilateral treaties on drug control and extended the existing control systems to include the cultivation of plants that were grown as the raw material of narcotic drugs. The principal objectives of the Convention are to limit the possession, use, trade in, distribution, import, export, manufacture and production of drugs exclusively to medical and scientific purposes and to address drug trafficking through international cooperation to deter and discourage drug traffickers. The Convention also established the International Narcotics Control Board, merging the Permanent Central Board and the Drug Supervisory Board.

(International Narcotics Control Board 2009a)

International drug policy is strongly influenced by the view that the best approach to drugs(except alcohol and tobacco) is to prohibit their use and to attempt to prevent their production, distribution, and use. The International Narcotics Control Board (INCB) was established in 1968 in accordance with the Single Convention. The INCB, an independent and judicial monitoring agency, has a remit that includes the following:

> As regards the licit manufacture of, trade in and use of drugs, INCB endeavours, in cooperation with Governments, to ensure that adequate supplies of drugs are available for medical and scientific uses and that the diversion of drugs from licit sources to illicit channels does not occur. INCB also monitors Governments' control over chemicals used in the illicit manufacture of drugs and assists them in preventing the diversion of those chemicals into the illicit traffic.
>
> As regards the illicit manufacture of, trafficking in and use of drugs, INCB identifies weaknesses in national and international control systems and contributes to correcting such situations. INCB is also responsible for assessing chemicals used in the illicit manufacture of drugs, in order to determine whether they should be placed under international control.
>
> (International Narcotics Control Board 2009b)

Both the current system of drug control in general, and the INCB, have many detractors. A number of commentators view the INCB as being reactionary and ideological:

> Nearly 400 years after Galileo Galilei of Florence was arraigned and convicted of suspected heresy by the ten member congregation of the Holy Office (Inquisition), the International Narcotics Control Board (INCB) is similarly inserting itself into matters pertaining to innovations in health care and the public health response to addiction throughout the world. Like that early inquisition of 1663 that convicted Galileo of heresy for holding that the sun is the centre of the universe with the earth revolving around the sun (in contradiction of church doctrine at the time) the INCB and its thirteen-member panel, now rails against any evidence out of sync with the established doctrine of the war on drugs: particularly those innovations in public health called harm reduction.
>
> The latest healthcare and harm reduction practices to attract the ire of the INCB Inquisition are elements of Canada's most effective and innovative measures to minimize the harms of drugs in Vancouver–supervised injection facilities and, recently, the potential establishment of supervised inhalation rooms–along with the long established practice of providing safer mouthpieces for pulmonary inhalation in British Columbia. This is particularly significant as it comes in the midst of a crucial battle between municipal and provincial authorities in BC with the federal government in Ottawa, which seems determined to undermine all the most effective HR programs that are the result of years of steady local and governmental support in Vancouver and now threatens to derail all these programs and spread doubt about their usefulness despite the overwhelmingly positive findings of serious research.
>
> (Small and Drucker 2008, p.16)

The INCB is the last of the UN drug agencies to still prioritize abstinence-only ideology over evidence-based policies that have proven effective in reducing drug-related harms. Its recommendations regarding substitution treatment, cannabis policy, and harm reduction measures to reduce death, disease, crime and suffering are all at odds with both scientific evidence and evolving policies in many parts of the world.

Perhaps most stunning is the Board's failure to consider the crime, violence and corruption as well as over-incarceration and violations of human rights associated with the global drug prohibition regime.

(Nadlemann 2009)

The drug control system is based primarily upon a regime of prohibition and the INCB is an unaccountable group of so-called experts who enforce the most counterproductive aspects of the UN Conventions. It is the global prohibition that deregulates the drugs market and the perverse economics of prohibition turn vegetables into products worth more than their weight in gold. By refusing to recognise and make explicit these counterproductive effects, the Board is supporting the worldwide catastrophe that ensues.

The Board is complicit in gifting the illegal drug market to terror groups, paramilitaries and organised criminals, contributing to the political and economic destabilisation of producer and transit countries and putting millions at risk of contracting blood-borne viruses. The INCB and the UN Office on Drugs and Crime pose a greater threat to global well-being than drugs themselves.

(D. Kushlick, personal communication)

The United Nations Office on Drugs and Crime (UNODC) has vehemently defended its position against growing criticisms of current international control policies. This is exemplified by the following recent statement:

Of late, there has been a limited but growing chorus among politicians, the press, and even in public opinion saying: drug control is not working. The broadcasting volume is still rising and the message spreading. Much of this public debate is characterized by sweeping generalizations and simplistic solutions. Yet, the very heart of the discussion underlines the need to evaluate the effectiveness of the current approach. Having studied the issue on the basis of our data, UNODC has concluded that, while changes are needed, they should be in favour of different means to protect society against drugs, rather than by pursuing the different goal of abandoning such protection.

What's the repeal debate about?

Several arguments have been put forward in favour of repealing drug controls, based on (i) economic, (ii) health, and (iii) security grounds, and a combination thereof.

I. The economic argument for drug legalization says: legalize drugs, and generate tax income. This argument is gaining favour, as national administrations seek new sources of revenue during the current economic crisis. This legalize and tax argument is un-ethical and uneconomical. It proposes a perverse tax, generation upon generation, on marginalized cohorts (lost to addiction) to stimulate economic recovery. Are the partisans of this cause also in favour of legalizing and taxing other seemingly intractable crimes like human trafficking? Modern- day slaves (and there are millions of them) would surely generate good tax revenue to rescue failed banks. The economic argument is also based on poor fiscal logic: any reduction in the cost of drug control (due to lower law enforcement expenditure) will be offset by much higher expenditure on public health (due to the surge of drug consumption). The moral of the story: don't make wicked transactions legal just because they are hard to control.

II. Others have argued that, following legalization, a health threat (in the form of a drug epidemic) could be avoided by state regulation of the drug market. Again, this is naive and myopic. First, the tighter the controls (on anything), the bigger and the faster a parallel (criminal) market will emerge–thus invalidating the concept. Second, only a few (rich) countries could afford such elaborate controls. What about the rest (the majority) of humanity? Why unleash a drug epidemic in the developing world for the sake of libertarian arguments made by a pro-drug lobby that has the luxury of access to drug treatment? Drugs are not harmful because they are controlled–they are controlled because they are harmful; and they do harm whether the addict is rich and beautiful, or poor and marginalized. Drug statistics keep speaking loud and clear. Past runaway growth has flattened out and the drug crisis of the 1990s seems under control. This 2009 Report provides further evidence that drug cultivation (opium and coca) are flat or down. Most importantly, major markets for opiates (Europe and South East Asia), cocaine (North America), and cannabis (North America, Oceania and Europe) are in decline. The increase in consumption of synthetic stimulants, particularly in East Asia and the Middle East, is cause for concern, although use is declining in developed countries.

III. The most serious issue concerns organized crime. All market activity controlled by the authority generates parallel, illegal transactions, as stated above. Inevitably, drug controls have generated a criminal market of macro- economic dimensions that uses violence and corruption to mediate between demand and supply. Legalize drugs, and organized crime will lose its most profitable line of activity, critics therefore say.

Not so fast. UNODC is well aware of the threats posed by international drug mafias. Our estimates of the value of the drug market (in 2005) were ground-breaking. The Office was also first to ring the alarm bell on the threat of drug trafficking to countries in West and East Africa, the Caribbean, Central America and the Balkans. In doing so we have highlighted the security menace posed by organized crime, a matter now periodically addressed by the UN Security Council. Having started this drugs/crime debate, and having pondered it extensively, we have concluded that these drug related, organized crime arguments are valid. They must be addressed. I urge governments to recalibrate the policy mix, without delay, in the direction of more controls on crime, without fewer controls on drugs. In other words, while the crime argument is right, the conclusions reached by its proponents are flawed. Why? Because we are not count- ing beans here: we are counting lives. Economic policy is the art of counting beans (money) and handling trade-offs: inflation vs. employment, consumption vs. savings, internal vs. external balances. Lives are different. If we start trading them off, we end up violating somebody's human rights. There cannot be exchanges, no quid-pro-quos, when health and security are at stake: modern society must, and can, protect both these assets with unmitigated determination. I appeal to the heroic partisans of the human rights cause worldwide, to help UNODC promote the right to health of drug addicts: they must be assisted and reintegrated into society. Addiction is a health condition and those affected by it should not be imprisoned, shot-at or, as suggested by the proponent of this argument, traded off in order to reduce the security threat posed by international mafias. Of course, the latter must be addressed.

(United Nations Office on Drugs and Crime 2009a, p.1)

A recent comment on the ideological divide concerning drug control policy has been provided by one of the Report's authors, Mike Trace:

Of course, one of the main difficulties for governments and international agencies lies in acknowledging the failure or limited impact of policies and strategies that they have previously promoted with such enthusiasm. Almost every government in the world has to some extent over the last 40 years advised its citizens that a tough anti-drug stance, backed up by strong enforcement of laws prohibiting drug production, distribution and use, will eventually lead to victory in the 'war on drugs'. This is a very attractive political message–drugs cause harm, so we are tough on drugs. Of course, it is more difficult politically to acknowledge that the reality has proved more complex, that you have made little progress, and all indications are that governments indeed do not have the powers and levers to eliminate the illegal market. Faced with this reality, particularly in a highly sensitive and polarised area of policy, most politicians and diplomats will seek to minimise scrutiny and keep their heads down. This, with a few brave exceptions, is what we have witnessed in Vienna in recent months.

Admitting to limited success is also institutionally dangerous. Many major national and international institutions have enjoyed constantly increasing budgets on the back of promises to win the fight against drug production, trafficking and use. The obvious question arising from an acknowledgment of limited success is whether those budgets have given value for money, or whether they should be re-allocated…

It is clear that the international community is now divided on the best way to respond to the continuing existence of a massive illegal global drug market, that continues to affect the lives of hundreds of millions of people. An increasingly clear difference of perspective is emerging between those who support the stronger and more consistent implementation of the drug conventions–focusing on clear social disapproval, and strong law enforcement–and those who support a rebalancing of policy and programmes towards a health and social inclusion approach. These are perfectly valid debates, being conducted between governments, academics and civil society. It is important, therefore, that these debates take place within a spirit of objective enquiry, with evidence and arguments focused on the ultimate objective of maximising the health and welfare of mankind, instead of political and institutional short-term self-interest.

(Trace 2009, personal communication; International Drug Policy Consortium 2009)

What these organizations and individuals seem to be saying is that the polarized debate is unhelpful. Legalization may appear to be an attractive and strong move to sweep away the damage done by corruption and the criminal trade in drugs but the stakes are too high and the unintended consequences are too risky for any government or international agency to consider. The health and social consequences are, however, increasing in importance and cost to the many countries affected. A refocus on mitigating the damage done by drugs seems to be emerging. This might have an effect on drug consumption and therefore an indirect benefit for the economic damage but it might also have a benefit for the welfare of an individual involved with drug taking.

This is not new and most countries have at the basis of their response to drug use a policy on ways of managing drug users and supporting them in their attempts to resolve their complex problems.

Harm minimization

Harm minimization or harm reduction is designed to reduce the levels of adverse effects of drug use while not necessarily requiring a cessation of such use itself. The aim of this approach is the avoidance of problems or harm (Strang and Stimson 1990, O'Hare et al. 1992, Heather et al. 1993). Harm-minimization approaches can take many forms, including the provision of free condoms and clean injecting equipment for intravenous drug users and the provision of bleach to enable such people to sterilize their injecting equipment. In its broadest sense harm reduction includes opiate-substitute treatment, education about the dangers of drugs, and engagement with drugs users in programmes to reduce drug intake, avoid injecting, or work towards abstinence. Harm minimization is, therefore, a broad approach embracing any policy or intervention which will mitigate the damaging effects of drug taking. This essentially pragmatic approach has been criticized on the grounds that it amounts to 'going soft' on drugs, or that it condones drug use. In fact, there is strong evidence showing that harm minimization can be highly effective in reducing the damage (such as HIV and hepatitis B and C infections) associated with intravenous drug use.

In fact, policies to prohibit or eradicate drug use and harm minimization are not necessarily mutually exclusive, even though they may be uneasy bedfellows. The reality is that many counties have signed up to drug prohibition, but implement practical strategies, such as types of drug treatment, which are forms of harm minimization.

Legalization

There is, of course another view. It is sometimes argued that drug use is inevitable and that most of the problems associated with it are due not to drug chemistry so much as the draconian social and legal response to drugs. This has forced drug use underground, created a vast criminal empire with drug lords, crime cartels, drug dealers, and a chronic international crime epidemic. However, it is not easy to have a rational debate about the legalization of drugs.

The global drug policy war

The international approach to drug policy has long been strongly influenced by the USA. The latter, pursuing its so-called War on Drugs, has sometimes insulted or bullied other countries (such as the Netherlands) that have opted for an approach based on harm reduction or harm minimization. One remarkable example of this was provided by General Barry McCafferty, then US Drug Tsar, in 1998. He wrongly claimed that the Dutch had a much higher murder rate than the USA, and attributed this 'fact' to drugs. In fact, the USA's murder rate at the time was more than four times that prevailing in the Netherlands. As noted by Garretsen (2009), the Dutch have recently been retreating from some of their better-known distinctive liberal policies in a mood of growing conservatism. An example of the strong influence of the USA has been provided by the suppression of a 1995 report by the World Health Organization (WHO). This was produced in the form of a briefing kit on global cocaine use. The text of this report (which remains unpublished) noted that the health problems associated with alcohol and tobacco use are far more widespread than those associated with cocaine. Moreover, the report was highly critical of US drug policy, suggesting that:

> supply reduction and law enforcement strategies have failed, and that options such as decriminalisation might be explored, flagging up such programmes in Australia, Bolivia, Canada and Colombia.

> (Goldacre 2009, p.8)

The report also stated that not all drug use is harmful and that occasional cocaine use does not appear to cause health or social problems. In addition, it maintained:

> Use of coca leaves appears to have no negative health effects and has positive, therapeutic, sacred and social functions for indigenous Andean populations.

> (Goldacre 2009, p.8)

These sentiments were heresy to the official US hard line on drugs and drug use. The report was not published because, as reported by Goldacre, the USA's representative to the WHO threatened to withdraw US financial support for the organization's research projects if it was. Goldacre has made the following comment on these events:

> In the case of cocaine there is an even more striking precedent for evidence being ignored: the World Health Organization (WHO) conducted what is probably the

largest ever study of global use. In March 1995 they released a briefing kit which summarised their conclusions, with some tantalising bullet points.

"Health problems from the use of legal substances, particularly alcohol and tobacco, are greater than health problems from cocaine use," they said. "Cocaine-related problems are widely perceived to be more common and more severe for intensive, high-dosage users and very rare and much less severe for occasional, low-dosage users."

The full report–which has never been published–was extremely critical of most US policies. It suggested that supply reduction and law enforcement strategies have failed, and that options such as decriminalisation might be explored, flagging up such programmes in Australia, Bolivia, Canada and Colombia. "Approaches which overemphasise punitive drug control measures may actually contribute to the development of heath-related problems," it said, before committing heresy by recommending research into the adverse consequences of prohibition, and discussing "harm reduction" strategies.

"An increase in the adoption of responses such as education, treatment and rehabilitation programmes," it said, "is a desirable counterbalance to the over-reliance on law enforcement."

It singled out anti-drug adverts based on fear. "Most programmes do not prevent myths, but perpetuate stereotypes and misinform the general public.

"Such programmes rely on sensationalised, exaggerated statements about cocaine which misinform about patterns of use, stigmatise users, and destroy the educator's credibility."

It also dared to challenge the prevailing policy view that all drug use is harmful misuse. "An enormous variety was found in the types of people who use cocaine, the amount of drug used, the frequency of use, the duration and intensity of use, the reasons for using and any associated problems."

Experimental and occasional use were by far the most common types of use, it said, and compulsive or dysfunctional use, though worthy of close attention, were much less common.

It then descended into outright heresy. "Occasional cocaine use does not typically lead to severe or even minor physical or social problems ... a minority of people ... use casually for a short or long period, and suffer little or no negative consequences."

And finally: "Use of coca leaves appears to have no negative health effects and has positive, therapeutic, sacred and social functions for indigenous Andean populations."

At the point where mild cocaine use was described in positive tones the Americans presumably blew some kind of outrage fuse. This report was never published because the US representative to the WHO threatened to withdraw US funding for all its research projects and interventions unless the organisation "dissociated itself from the study" and cancelled publication. According to the WHO this document does not exist (although you can read a leaked copy at www.tdpf.org.uk/WHOleaked.pdf).

Drugs show the classic problem for evidence-based social policy. It may well be that prohibition, and distribution of drugs by criminals, gives worse results for the outcomes we think are important, such as harm to the user and to communities through crime. But equally, we may tolerate these outcomes, because we decide it is more important that we declare ourselves to disapprove of drug use. It's okay to do that.

> You can have policies that go against your stated outcomes, for moral or political reasons: but that doesn't mean you can hide the evidence.
>
> (Goldacre 2009, p.8)

It has been reported that, even with the accession of President Barack Obama's more liberal administration in 2009, the USA was continuing to criticize the European Union's harm-reduction approach to drugs. The latter supports needle-and-syringe exchanges (Campbell and Hirsch 2009).

The drug marketplace is worldwide in its scope. Some drug traffickers have vast wealth, together with tame political and military protectors, fleets of motor vehicles, high speed boats, ships, aircraft, and even submarines (Thompson 2007, Oobject 2008). Many areas of the world, including South and Central America, parts of Africa, and Asia are in turmoil because of illicit drugs. They generate vast wealth for some, but also cause political and social chaos on a horrifying scale. The latter is exemplified by the fact that in Mexico, for example, thousands of people are dying each year in violence between the authorities and drug traffickers and conflict between members of rival drug cartels.

The War on Drugs has not been going well. Some international policies, such as forcible crop eradication in countries such as Afghanistan and Colombia, are morally suspect and sometimes completely counterproductive. In fact the War on Drugs is linked to another global conflict, the post-11 September 2001 ('9/11') War on Terror or so-called Long War (Tisdall and MacAskill 2006). It has been widely reported that the drug trade plays a significant role in many recent and contemporary political and military upheavals:

> There is evidence that many terrorist organizations and some rogue regimes pressed for cash rely on the illicit drug trade as a source of income. In the case of Afghanistan, reports indicating that the drug trade is a major source of income for the Taliban have received growing attention. According to some reports, the regime uses poppy-derived income to arm, train and support fundamentalist groups including the Islamic Movement of Uzbekistan (IMU) and the Chechen resistance. There have also been allegations of Osama bin Laden's personal involvement in drug trafficking to finance al Qaeda's activities.
>
> (Perle 2001)

This quotation is hardly from a neutral source. Even so, it does point to the undeniable linkages between drug production and political unrest. Just imagine, your country is invaded by foreigners and many of your traditional crops are 'eradicated' by the invaders' superior military forces. The latter justify this because they view your main cash crops as being harmful. 'Shock and awe' are followed by hatred. Sadly, such events have been the recent experience in several countries. In 2007 Simon Jenkins scathingly described the situation in Afghanistan's Helmand Province thus:

> Poppy production in Afghanistan has soared since the invasion, this year alone by 34%. The harvest in the British-occupied protectorate of Helmand rose by 50% in 12 months. This is a dazzling triumph for agricultural intervention.
>
> Ministers may deny that this was their policy, but they cannot be that inept. They faced a heroin epidemic at home. Suddenly finding themselves charged with controlling almost all the world's opium production, they must have known what they were doing. By alienating farmers and forcing them into the arms of the Taliban, they would drive up illicit production, and encourage oversupply.

(Jenkins 2007, p.29)

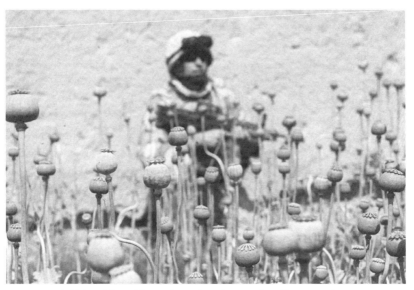

A British soldier of Second Royal Regiment of Fusiliers patrols near a poppy field in the Sangin district of Afghanistan

Credit: AP/Press Association Images.

One factor that further complicates the changing drug situation in Afghanistan is the fact that many of the national police use drugs:

> Of 5,320 Afghan police and recruits tested by US-led police training programmes across the country, 16% were found to be using drugs. The majority of those who tested positive had used cannabis or opium.
>
> Analysts say that the drug problem in the police is higher in the southern provinces where drugs are readily available - in Kandahar province, which neighbours Helmand, 38% tested positive.
>
> Police work in these areas is also highly dangerous and low paid - reasons, analysts say, for widespread drug use.

"The police are constantly under threat from the Taleban," says Abdul Ghafoor, director of the Regional Studies Centre of Afghanistan, a think-tank based in Kabul.
"To escape from the psychological pressure they often turn to drugs."
But Mr Ghafoor insists that it is vital for Afghanistan that the police act within the law.
"The police are responsible for controlling drug trafficking, but if they become addicts who will control it?"

(Patience 2009)

The UNODC reported in August 2008 that, while overall opium production in Afghanistan had fallen in the past year, in several provinces (including Helmand, producing 75% of the national total) it had continued to rise. It was also noted that one of the main beneficiaries of opium sales was the Taliban. It was reported that the Taliban obtained £50 000 000 from opium sales in 2007 (BBC News Online, 24 June, 2008b, United Nations News Centre 2008). In its most recent Afghan Opium Survey, the UNODC (United Nations Office on Drugs and Crime 2009b) reported (at the time this book was being written) that there had been a further 10% fall in Afghan poppy production. The United Nations attributed this drop to vigorous anti-drug activity by NATO and Afghan armed forces. They noted that 20 out of 34 provinces appeared to be 'poppy-free'. Moreover, the biggest fall in poppy cultivation had been evident in the war-torn southern province of Helmand, where poppy cultivation had fallen by 30%. This success was partly attributed to the promotion of other types of (legal) agriculture.

A report by BBC Scotland reported that 90% of the UK's heroin originates from Afghan opium poppies (Bird 2008). It has also been reported that:

A form of high grade white heroin is making a comeback in the UK, despite having virtually disappeared during the 1980s and 90s, officials have said.

(BBC News Online, 1 February, 2009a)

This heroin, it has been claimed, originates from Afghanistan.

The situation in most parts of Afghanistan, teetering on the brink of becoming a 'failed state', is dire. Western policy is clearly not working as intended. Seymour Hersh (2005) cites a non-governmental organization (NGO) official who claimed that: 'Everybody knows that the U.S. Military has the drug lords on the payroll. We've put them back in power. It's all gone terribly wrong'.

The Senlis Council produced a report, *Stumbling into Chaos: Afghanistan on the Brink,* on the escalating production of Afghan opium in 2007. This recommended buying up the entire crop (Senlis Council 2007). This report was poorly received by agencies such as the UK Government, NATO, and the United Nations. Curiously, it became evident during 2008 that some Afghan farmers had abandoned growing poppies. This change was not caused by drug control policies. The growing world food shortage—partly due to a switch by some farmers from food production to biofuel production—has inflated the price of wheat, making it a far more attractive crop:

> Market forces have been the deciding factor – with wheat prices doubling in the past year, and the street price of heroin falling, it is now more cost effective to grow wheat.

> (Coughlin 2008)

In spite of this, reports in mid-2008 suggested that the Taliban insurgents were still increasing their profits from opium production. One recent bizarre suggestion is that Afghan poppy cultivation should be boosted even more in order to depress prices and flood the market. Such a step might threaten to channel surplus drugs into Iran and China, both of which already have huge addict populations.

In August 2009 a report by the House of Commons Foreign Affairs Committee was published. This acknowledged that Afghanistan was 'a poisoned chalice' and that the UK was failing to meet its objectives there. A major reason for this, the Committee members claimed, was 'mission creep': the UK and its forces had taken on too any objectives, including the suppression of the illegal drug trade. The committee recommended that British armed forces should withdraw from drug enforcement, leaving this to other agencies such as the Afghan army.

Colombia, long notorious for being a 'narco state', has played a massive role in the industrial-scale production of cocaine. During their heyday, the notorious Medellín Cartel was believed to earn US$30 billion a year from cocaine trading. At one stage it was credited with controlling 80% of the world's supply of cocaine. The ruthless and violent drug lord Pablo Escobar, rated the seventh richest man in the world, offered to pay off Colombia's national debt in 1984 to avoid extradition to the USA. At one stage the Colombian Government confiscated 300 light aircraft from cartel members (Bowden 2001, Escobar 2009). It has even been suggested that during the 2008/9 world financial crisis some international banks only avoided collapse thanks to the fact that drug money kept them afloat (Syal 2009).

Colombia has been torn by internecine conflict between Marxist guerillas, rightwing paramilitary groups, and drug lords for decades. It has been teetering on the brink of becoming a lawless and chaotic failed state, like Somalia. The British Royal Navy has been active and successful in seizing huge amounts of illicit drugs in the Caribbean as well as in other areas. These seizures included a single consignment of over 5 tons of cocaine worth over £240 000 000.

The UNODC has recently reported that the global picture was far from encouraging:

> The long-term stabilization of world drug markets continued into 2007, although notable exceptions occurred in some critical areas. As long term trends are obviously more meaningful and indicative than short term fluctuations, these limited reversals do not appear to negate the containment of the drug markets recorded since the late 1990s.
>
> On the supply side, despite cultivation increases for both coca and opiates in 2007, the overall level of cultivation remained below the one recorded at the beginning of the UNGASS [UN General Assembly Special Session on Drugs] process (1998) and well below annual peaks in the last two decades (1991 for opium and 2000 for coca). In 2007, opium cultivation increased in both Afghanistan and Myanmar: coupled with higher yields, especially in southern Afghanistan, this generated much greater world output. With regard to cocaine, cultivation increased in Bolivia, Peru and especially Colombia, but yields declined, so production remained stable. On the demand side, despite an apparent increase in the absolute number of cannabis, cocaine and opiates users, annual prevalence levels have remained stable in all drug markets. In other words, as the number of people who have used a particular drug at least once in the past 12 months has risen at about the same rate as population, drug consumption has remained stable in relative terms. Given these yearly changes, the containment of world drug markets – recorded in these reports over the last few years – appears confirmed but under strain. Further consolidation, in 2008 and beyond, will mean tightening overall market containment and addressing slippage in areas where some expansion was registered in 2007. On the supply side this dictates two critical priorities: lowering opium poppy cultivation, especially in Afghanistan; and returning to the path of steadily declining coca cultivation registered in the first few years of this century. On the demand side, more effectively containing the number of drug users, particularly in developing countries, has to become a critical priority; and more attention should be given to prevention, treatment and reducing the negative consequences of drug abuse. Rich countries' drugs markets fluctuate, mostly sideways and occasionally downwards: it is equally important to nurture and fortify the downward trend.
>
> The containment of illicit drug use to less than 5% of the world population aged 15 to 64 (based on annual prevalence estimates…is a considerable achievement…)

(United Nations Office on Drugs and Crime 2008, p.7)

The UK: drug policy and drug rhetoric

Reports on UK drug policy

This book cannot do justice to all of the lengthy discussions that have taken place into UK drug policy in recent years. As noted above, these discussions have included several very weighty reports. Several of these have concluded that there are major limitations in current UK drug policy and that some major changes are required. It is worthwhile to cite some of these documents in brief: It is hoped that this will provide at least a superficial insight into the format and main conclusions of these reports. It is, however, strongly recommended that people who are interested should read the originals in full.

Police Foundation (2000) *Drugs and the Law: Report of the Independent Inquiry into the Misuse of Drugs Act 1971* (the Runciman Report)

This heavyweight report has provided a detailed and authoritative critique of the Misuse Drugs Act (1971). This report set out to consider what social changes had occurred since the introduction of the Act. It also sought to evaluate the degree to which the law needed revision to make it more effective and responsive to social change. The report included the conclusion that the eradication of drug use was unattainable and that it was far more realistic for the law to seek to: 'control and limit the demand for and the supply of illicit drugs in order to minimize the serious individual and social harms caused by their use'. The report, a very thoughtful document, drew attention to the fact that there was a weak evidence base and little UK research. This included no real early-warning system to detect new changes in drug use such as those developed in the Netherlands and the USA. The report's authors conclude that existing UK drug policy appeared to have only a limited deterrent effect and that both casual and problem drug use had increased during the past 30 years. They noted that there appeared to be up to 200 000 problem drug users, most of whom were heroin users and that such problem use was associated with social deprivation. The committee concluded that the perceived health risks of drug use appeared to be more of a deterrent to drug use than the fact that such substances were illegal. The committee pointed out that although the UK was bound by international drug-control obligations, there was some scope for amending some aspects of the drug control law. They went on to recommend the reclassification of several drugs. These were cannabis (from Category B to Category C), ecstasy and LSD (from A to B), cannabinol and its derivatives (from A to C), and a semi-synthetic opiate called buprenorphine (Temgesic) from C to B.

Beckley Foundation (2005) *Facing the Future: The Challenge for National & International Drug Policy*

This report by the Beckley Foundation is one of several that have concluded that current UK and international drug polices have not been very effective. The authors point out that as the network of drug-control policies has been extended, drug use has continued to increase. They succinctly detail the harms associated both with drug use and with current 'zero-tolerance' approaches that attempt to control it. They note that they were unable to find any convincing example of successful supply reduction, nor any 'clear links' between law enforcement and the supply of drugs on the street. They did, however, acknowledge that:

> Successful examples of supply reduction were either for particular drugs only (for example in Australia, where we found evidence of dependent users switching to other drugs) and/or comparatively short-lived (for example Australia and Thailand), and/ or achieved at an unacceptable cost in terms of respect for judicial norms and violations of human rights (for example Thailand's 'war on drugs' or the Taliban in Afghanistan).
>
> (Beckley Foundation 2005, p.3)

They suggest that, in view of the failure of existing control policies, 'a new global drug policy paradigm' is required. The report recommends that national drug policies should not suggest that they will achieve 'sharp reductions' in drug use, since this is unrealistic. They also recommend not spending most of the available resources on drug enforcement, but rather on demand reduction and harm minimization. They conclude that drug policies should adhere to the following standards:

1 the guiding principle for international drug policy should be to reduce drug-related harm;
2 the principal harms are crime and public nuisance, drug-related deaths, physical and mental health problems, social costs, and environmental damage;
3 the development of drug policy must be guided by evidence collection and evaluation, which is open to public scrutiny and informs periodic and objective policy review;
4 drug policy should respect human rights, local judicial norms, and divergent cultural attitudes to drugs and drug use.

Foresight (2007) *Drugs Futures 2025?* Foresight Drug Science, Addiction & Drugs Project

Drug researchers are familiar with the harsh reality that it is often hard to monitor and describe what has been happening. One recent enterprise set out to do something much harder, to contemplate what might happen in future. The Foresight project was conducted to answer the following multi-faceted question: how can we manage the use of psychoactive substances in the future to best advantage for the individual, the community, and society?

The background to this ambitious exercise was the fact that there have been major scientific advances in several disciplines which relate to the brain and human behaviour. It was decided to consider how such advances might be applied in the next 20 years in relation to mental health, the effects of legal and illicit drugs, and mental processes. It was concluded that: new drugs might help people to 'forget' addictions, vaccines may be developed to stop the action of addictive drugs on the brain, genomics might help treatments to be targeted more effectively, a drug has been found that can block the memory-impairing effects of alcohol in humans, and non-addictive recreational drugs may be produced which are less harmful than existing ones.

It should be emphasized that although these conclusions reflect recent scientific advances, some of them were at least partly speculative. The search for a problem-free recreational drug is akin to the addiction field's quest for the Holy Grail. This has been in unsuccessful progress for some time, with a number of false dawns (remember 'non-addictive' heroin and benzodiazepines?). The concept of a harm-free recreational drug is akin to *Star Trek*'s synthehol, tasting like alcohol but without any of its deleterious effects.

The report also speculated about the moral ethical and philosophical issues which would arise in a situation where happiness might be achieved by use of a safe and effective medicine without side effects.

Royal Society for the Encouragement of Arts, Manufactures and Commerce (2007) *Drugs-Facing Facts*

The Royal Society for the Encouragement of Arts, Manufactures and Commerce (RSA) Commission on Illegal Drugs, Communities and Public Policy has produced a wide-ranging and very thoughtful and thorough overview of drug use in the UK. This includes a succinct review of drug effects, drug policy development, policy options, and approaches to improving treatment and support for those with drug-related problems. The report concludes that drug use is probably inevitable and that the concept of a drug-free Britain is a 'chimera'. Since this term refers to an animal hybrid consisting of two or more unrelated species the meaning of this pronouncement is unclear. Even so, the report makes it clear that its authors regard drug use as being here to stay. They make the point that illicit drug use has been demonized in ways that alcohol and tobacco have not. A 'calm, rational and balanced' approach would be preferable. Yes it would! The report concludes that drug markets cannot simply be closed down. They are too resilient for that. It also concluded that illicit drug use is evident throughout the country and in all socio-economic groups. Moreover, most drug users do not appear to be damaged by their use. Drug use is, however, associated with mental health problems, premature mortality, and crime. The committee recommended that illicit drugs should be brought under a single regulatory framework along with alcohol and tobacco. They acknowledge that the UK's mainly crime-prevention/criminal justice approach to drug use has not been very successful. They appeal for a more 'holistic' system, incorporating a rejection of the assumption that having prohibition as its main goal can work. The committee appealed for a major revision of the Government's National Drug Strategy:

> Drugs policy should be better integrated into policies in such areas as social exclusion, housing and homelessness and regeneration, just as they are increasingly being integrated into policies on children and young people.
>
> (Royal Society for the Encouragement of Arts, Manufactures and Commerce 2007, p.17)

Two of the most significant recommendations of the committee were, firstly, that future drug policy, like that related to alcohol and tobacco, should be designed not to eradicate use, but to regulate use and prevent harm, and secondly that the remit of the Advisory Council on the Misuse of Drugs should be extended to cover alcohol and tobacco.

Scotland's Futures Forum (2008) *Approaches to Alcohol and Drugs in Scotland: A Question of Architecture*

This report was produced to determine how the damage caused by alcohol and illicit drug use could be halved by the year 2025. The study involved consultations with a wide variety of people, including academics, young people, service users, and the parents of problems drug users, together with people working in the health and social services and industry. A systems mapping approach was used in relation to a review of seven areas. These were the culture of substance use, governance, enforcement, treatment interventions and recovery support, public health, community level factors, and evidence and research. The report, which includes some rather labyrinthine diagrams, concludes that it might be possible to reduce the level of alcohol and drug-related harm in Scotland by action targeted in the seven domains that were identified. This would involve steps such as basing policy on evidence and research, to strengthen 'the preventive and supportive capacity of local communities, including reducing inequality....' The report concedes that alcohol and drug use provide a complex challenge for policy makers. This was the reason for using the systems mapping approach, since this takes account of the complexities and contradictions which bedevil topics such as drug problems. It goes on the note that:

> A unifying framework of theory and practices on the use of alcohol, tobacco and other substances will be necessary if we are to achieve a significant reduction in damage by 2025. Action, however, in many areas must be taken in the near future as well as the medium and long term.... The challenge to reduce alcohol and drug damage by half is manageable if there is willingness to use current understanding of what is effective.
>
> (Scotland's Futures Forum 2008, p.14)

UK Drug Policy Commission (2008) *Reducing Drug Use, Reducing Reoffending: are Programmes for Problem Drug-using Offenders in the UK Supported by the Evidence?*

The UK Drug Policy Commission produced another well-argued report in 2008. Like the earlier report by the Police Foundation (2000), this was produced by a committee chaired by Dame Ruth Runciman, a past member of the Advisory Council on the Misuse of Drugs and former Chair of the UK Mental Health Commission.

This report identified its focus as examining the evidence for the effectiveness of initiatives to provide treatment and support services for drug-dependent offenders. In particular, the committee sought to analyse evidence that this approach had succeeded in reducing drug use and reoffending as part of a more general appraisal of the criminal justice approach to illicit drug use. The report provided details of the massive scale of drug-related offending. This included the fact that:

> at least 1 in 8 arrestees (equivalent to about 125,000 people in England and Wales) are estimated to be problem heroin and/or crack users, compared with about 1 in 100 of the gereral population.... Between a third and a half of new receptions to prison are estimated to be problem drug users…
>
> (UK Drug Policy Commission 2008, p.7)

The committee noted that there was a wide and complex array of interventions operating to identify drug using offenders, and to encourage them to contact treatment and support services, both in the community and within the criminal justice system. They concluded that they were unable to assess the overall impact of using the criminal justice system to manage problem drug use. It was concluded that some evidence supported drug courts, community sentences, prison-based therapeutic communities, opioid detoxification, and methadone maintenance with prison and the community, and the RAP-12 Step abstinence-based programme. Overall, the committee concluded that evidence on impact of the criminal justice approach was patchy. It was not clear which modes of help/support were best for which people. Even so, more research was needed to improve the evidence base about the effectiveness of policy options. Moreover, it was, they believed, justified to use criminal-justice-based interventions to encourage problem drug users to engage with treatment programmes.

The recent drug debate

The debate about drugs and drug policy can get very nasty. People who advocate the legalization of all drugs run the risk of being ridiculed or vilified by most politicians and, not least, by the notorious British 'red-top' or tabloid press. This has been exemplified by the generally hostile response to comments by Mr Richard Brunstrom, Chief Constable of North Wales, reported here in the broadsheet newspaper, *The Independent*:

> One of Britain's most senior police officers is to call for all drugs–including heroin and cocaine–to be legalised and urges the Government to declare an end to the "failed" war on illegal narcotics.
>
> Richard Brunstrom, the Chief Constable of North Wales, advocates an end to UK drug policy based on "prohibition". His comments come as the Home Office this week ends the process of gathering expert advice looking at the next 10 years of strategy.
>
> In his radical analysis, which he will present to the North Wales Police Authority today, Mr Brunstrom points out that illegal drugs are now cheaper and more plentiful than ever before.
>
> The number of users has soared while drug-related crime is rising with narcotics now supporting a worldwide business empire second only in value to oil. "If policy on drugs is in future to be pragmatic not moralistic, driven by ethics not dogma, then the current prohibitionist stance will have to be swept away as both unworkable and immoral, to be replaced with an evidence-based unified system (specifically including tobacco and alcohol) aimed at minimisation of harms to society," he will say.
>
> The demand will not find favour in Downing Street. In his conference speech this year, Gordon Brown signalled an intensification of the existing battle. 'We will send out a clear message that drugs are never going to be decriminalized', the Prime Minister told the party.
>
> The Tories also rejected the proposals. David Davis, the shadow Home Secretary, said a more effective move would be the creation of a UK border police force to stop drugs getting into the country as well as expanding rehabilitation centres. He added: 'We would put police on the streets to catch and deter drug dealers and we would ensure sufficient prison capacity so they could actually be punished'.
>
> Mr Brunstrom, whose championing of speed cameras has made him a hate figure among some motoring groups, also found his suggestion that the war on drugs was unwinnable dismissed as a 'counsel of despair' by the Association of Chief Police Officers (ACPO). 'Moving to total legalization would, in our view, greatly exacerbate the harm to people in this country, not reduce it', an ACPO spokeswoman said.
>
> But the 30-page report, entitled Drugs Policy–a radical look ahead, includes a number of persuasive voices. Today Mr Brunstrom will urge his colleagues to submit the paper to Westminster and the Welsh Assembly. In it, he quotes the findings in March this year of a Royal Society for the Encouragement of Arts commission, which stated that 'the law as it stands is not fit for purpose' and argues for the replacement of the 1971 Misuse of Drugs Act with a new Misuse of Substances Act.
>
> That would mean scrapping the ABC system introduced by the Home Secretary James Callaghan with a new scale that assesses substances, including alcohol and tobacco, in relation to the harm they cause–although he admits banning booze and cigarettes is not likely.
>
> But he notes that figures from the Chief Medical Officer have found that, in Scotland, 13 000 people died from tobacco-related use in 2004 while 2,052 died as a result of alcohol. Illegal drugs, meanwhile, accounted for 356 deaths. The maximum

penalty for possessing a class A drug is 14 years in prison while supplying it carries a life term.

Mr Brunstrom indicates that there is a growing mood for change. He cites the House of Commons Select Committee on Science and Technology, which criticized the Government for failing to switch to an evidence-based policy approach. The report also includes quotes from former home secretary John Reid, admitting 'prohibition' doesn't work, and the Olympics minister, Tessa Jowell, conceding 'it drives the activity underground'. There is also supportive evidence from former Chief Inspector of Prisons Lord Ramsbotham, a retired High Court judge, and Scotland's Drug Tsar, Tom Wood.

As well as hitting the country hard in economic terms – class A drug use in England and Wales costs the country up to £17bn a year, 90 per cent of which is due to crime–there are also a series of socially damaging knock-on effects, he says.

He argues that prohibition has created a crisis in the criminal justice system, destabilized producer countries and undermined human rights worldwide. By pursuing a policy of legalization and regulation, he concludes, the Government will 'dramatically reduce drug-related criminality and will enable significant funds to be transferred from law enforcement to harm reduction and treatment procedures that are known to work'.

There was a mixed response from groups that work with users. Danny Kushlick, a director of the charity Transform Drug Policy Foundation, praised Mr Brunstrom for his 'great leadership and imagination'. But Clare McNeil, a policy officer for Addaction, said talk of legalization distracted attention from the more important issue of rehabilitation. 'We have some sympathy with his views and the reasons and why he believes this but we are not in favour of legalization', she said.

Nick Clegg, the Liberal Democrat home affairs spokesman, said it was 'significant' that a senior police officer had spoken out although he too thought the police chief's views went too far. 'Where he is absolutely right is that the Government's drugs policy is failing and failing spectacularly. The refusal of the Government to think radically means we are letting thousands of young boys and girls down.

'I am not persuaded that full legalization is the way forward but what is necessary is that a more logical and evidence-based approach is needed which is less susceptible to whims of individual home secretaries . . . The system does not work as it is'.

The Chief Constable's verdict

British drugs policy has been based upon prohibition for the last several decades–but this system has not worked well. Illegal drugs are in plentiful supply and have become consistently cheaper in real terms over the years.

The number of drug users has increased dramatically. Drug-related crime has soared equally sharply as a direct consequence of the illegality of some drugs. The vast profits from illegal trading have supported a massive rise in organized crime.

Mr Brunstrom says: 'If policy on drugs is in the future to be pragmatic not moralistic, driven by ethics not dogma, then the current prohibitionist stance will have to be swept away as both unworkable and immoral. Such a strategy leads inevitably to the legalization and regulation of all drugs'.

The chief constable asserts that current British drugs policy is based upon an unwinnable 'war on drugs' enshrined in a flawed understanding of the underlying United

Nations conventions, and arising from a wholly outdated and thoroughly repugnant moralistic stance.

He concludes: "The law is the law. In the meantime, I will continue to enforce it to the best of my ability despite my misgivings about its moral and practical worth."

(Brown and Langton 2007)

Mr Brunstrom's views were given further support by a former chief inspector of prisons:

Lord Ramsbotham argued that the huge number of people in jail with a drug problem proved that current policy, based on "prohibition", was not working. Richard Brunstrom, the Chief Constable of North Wales, provoked controversy after he said the "war on drugs" could not be won and should be replaced with a radical new approach. Lord Ramsbotham said: "The present regime has failed in every way. If you look at prohibition of alcohol in the US, it failed. The Chief Constable's suggestions must be considered seriously. We've got to stop the dealers who cause so much misery for society.

(Morris 2007)

The *Daily Mail*, always ready to add an enlightened, dignified comment on any important social issue, called Mr Brunstrom 'the most idiotic police Chief in Britain'. This accolade was prompted by his advocacy of drug legalization and his comments to the effect that ecstasy was a relatively safe drug (Daily Mail 2007). In fact, Richard Bruntrom is by no means the first senior police officer to advocate a different approach to drugs:

Police officers are calling for all drugs to be legalised in Scotland. In a hugely controversial move, an influential group of frontline officers is demanding a radical change in the law. They say that even Class A drugs such as cocaine and heroin should no longer be illegal. The call comes from rank and file police in the country's biggest force who say radical measures are essential to tackle the spiralling drug problem.

Strathclyde Police Federation which represents nearly all 7,700 officers in the area, says all drugs should be licensed for use by addicts. The Association says millions of pounds are wasted on futile efforts to tackle the issue, with resources diverted from other police duties.

...

Inspector Jim Duffy, chairman of the federation, said the approach to drug abuse must be transformed in order to cut the death toll. He said:"We should legalise all drugs currently covered by the Misuse of Drugs Act–everything from class A to C, including heroin, cocaine and speed.

"We are not winning the war against drugs and we need to think about different ways to tackle it. Tell me a village where they are drug-free?"

He added: "Despite the amount of resources and the fantastic work our girls and guys do, we are not making a difference. We don't have any control at the moment.

Strathclyde Police Federation plans to table a discussion motion at the body's forthcoming national conference to garner support from officers across Scotland.

(Daily Mail Scotland 2006, p.1)

Another high-profile critic of the UK's current 'get tough' drug-enforcement policies spoke out in August 2008. Julian Critchley, the civil servant who had directed the cabinet's anti-drug unit, described current drug policies as being pointless and ineffective. He noted that the UK drugs market was saturated and that people could obtain any illicit drugs they wanted without difficulty:

> The idea that many people are holding back solely because of a law which they know is already unenforceable is simply ridiculous…. The argument is always put forward against this (legalisation) is that there would be a commensurate increase in drug use as the result of legalisation…. This, it seems to me is a bogus point: tobacco is a legal drug, whose use is declining, and precisely because it is legal, its users are far more amenable to government control, education programmes and taxation than they would be were it illegal.

> (BBC News Online, 13 August, 2008c)

The response from the Daily Mail, dependably hostile to any relaxing of strict drug controls, was to note that:

> senior MPs, police chiefs and anti-narcotics campaigners lined up to condemn him as 'utterly irresponsible.'

> (Drury 2008)

Reclassify all drugs?

There has long been disagreement about what some view as the arbitrary nature of the existing system of drug classification under the Misuse of Drugs Act. A report from the Science and Technology Committee of the House of Commons had reached the following conclusion:

> With respect to the ABC classification system, we have identified significant anomalies in the classification of individual drugs and a regrettable lack of consistency in the rationale used to make classification decisions. In addition, we have expressed concern at the Government's proclivity for using the classification system as a means of 'sending out signals' to potential users and society at large—it is at odds with the stated objective of classifying drugs on the basis of harm and the Government has not made any attempt to develop an evidence base on which to draw in determining the 'signal' being sent out.

> (Science and Technology Committee 2006)

A review by Professor David Nutt (who gave evidence to the above committee) and colleagues concluded that there was a more rational way of classifying overall drug dangers. This is considered further in Chapter 8.

> A law banning magic mushrooms and making them a class A drug has come into force. The Drugs Act 2005 ends the situation in which fresh magic mushrooms were legal but those which were dried or prepared for use were not. Sellers have condemned

the move, saying mushrooms are not harmful and accusing ministers of a knee-jerk reaction.

But the Home Office said the drug was harmful to some users and added the move clarified the existing law. Home Office Minister Paul Goggins said in a statement: "Magic mushrooms are a powerful hallucinogen and can cause real harm, especially to vulnerable people and those with mental health problems."

(BBC News Online, 18 July, 2005)

The UK, like most countries, is bound by international treaties related to drug control. These include the Single Convention on Narcotic Drugs (1961), the Convention on Psychotropic Substances (1971), and the Convention against the Illicit Traffic in Narcotic Drugs and Psychotropic Substances (1988). These treaties will be described and their implications will be considered. In particular the conflict between drug-enforcement strategies (such as criminalizing drug use and crop eradication) and harm minimization will be considered. British drug policies (including the former UK Labour government's 10-year drug strategy: see below) will be critically examined. It will be noted that both national and international policies have fallen hugely short of their goal of achieving a substantial reduction in either the use of illicit drugs or the adverse consequences of such use.

Drug policies

There is no shortage of drug policy statements. The European Union (EU) had a Drugs Action Plan covering the period 2005–8. This was part of a broader EU Drug Strategy (2005–12). These policies include the challenging areas of demand and supply reduction. As noted by the European Monitoring Centre for Drugs and Drug Addiction (EMCDDA), EU policy listed approximately 100 specific actions that were due to be assessed by 2008. A second action plan is planned to cover the period 2009–12 (EMCDDA 2009a). The number of national drug policy documents has proliferated in recent years. It has recently been noted that all EU member states apart from Austria have such policies. In the case of Austria, policies do exist, but relate to separate provinces (EMCDDA 2008).

Current policies in the UK

As noted by Reuter and Stevens (2007), the administrations of the devolved components of the UK have been active in formulating drug policy statements. These are all in many respects praiseworthy. They include much the same ingredients, but the latter are presented in varied ways and with a differing emphasis. The former UK Labour government's 10-year drug strategy,

Tackling Drugs to Build a Better Britain, was published in 1998. This set out the following four objectives:

> Young People – to help young people resist drug misuse in order to achieve their full potential in society;
> Communities – to protect our communities from drug-related anti-social and criminal behaviour;
> Treatment – to enable people with drug problems to overcome them and live healthy and crime-free lives;
> Availability – to stifle the availability of illegal drugs on our streets.

(President of the Council 1998, p.1)

This document was elaborated 4 years later by the *Updated Drug Strategy* (Home Office 2002). This provided more emphasis on Class A drugs and their users, the use of police hit squads to target 'middle drug markets', better targeting of the communities most affected by drugs, the expansion of treatment services, drug education, support for parents, carers and families, expanded outreach for vulnerable young people, and aftercare and 'throughfare' services to improve access to treatment and to reduce the chances of ex-prisoners reoffending or relapsing into drug addiction. The drug strategy had enabled the government, it claimed, to achieve a reduction in drug-related crime, and associated harm as well as raising the numbers of offenders receiving treatment.

A new drug strategy for England and Wales was announced in 2008 (HM Government 2008a). Like its widely criticized predecessor, this strategy gives heavy emphasis to drug prohibition. Its main focus was on the connection between certain types of drug use (such as crack and heroin) and crime:

> The drug strategy aims to restrict the supply of illegal drugs and reduce the demand for them. It focuses on protecting families and strengthening communities.
> The four main strands of work are:
> protecting communities through robust enforcement to tackle drug supply, drug-related crime and anti-social behaviour preventing harm to children, young people and families affected by drug misuse delivering new approaches to drug treatment and social re-integration public information campaigns, communications and community engagement.

(HM Government 2008a)

The new strategy, the government noted, was underpinned by a series of 3-year action plans, starting with *Drugs: Protecting Families and Communities. Action plan 2008-2011* (HM Government 2008b). The plan outlined a series of objectives, actions, and outcomes under four main strands of work. One area is the further development of the FRANK drugs-education campaign to be achieved, it was stated, among other ways, through the delivery of information on most commonly used drugs and by supporting stakeholders to deliver local information and prevention campaigns. This approach has the aim of increasing awareness of the risks of drug and alcohol use among young people and changing attitudes. The plan also highlights a drive towards providing advice and information to parents with the aim of increasing parental involvement to prevent drug taking in young people. The action plan identified a very large number of laudable components related to the criminal justice system, including law enforcement. These include improving joint working by prison and probation services, evaluating integrated offender management, improving accommodation and employment for ex-offenders, improving prison-based treatments, and reducing the supply of drugs in prison (and in Afghanistan). In addition, a number of objectives were identified relating to families, communities, and young people. These included encouraging work on families and drug use, fostering greater use of childcare, provision of treatment for drug-using parents, encouraging greater cooperation between treatment and maternity services, supporting drug-using parents, family self-help groups, carers, and providing and evaluating drug education.

The Scottish Drug Strategy, *The Road to Recovery: A New Approach to Tackling Scotland's Drug Problem*, was published in May 2008 (Scottish Government 2008). The tone and emphasis of the Scottish Government's strategy were rather different from the corresponding documents for England and Wales. The Scottish strategy focused far more on therapeutic issues (notably recovery) and was less dominated by heavy emphasis on the criminal justice system. Policies both north and south of Hadrian's Wall included a focus on prevention that did not appear to be unduly influenced by the fact that preventing drug use has a very poor track record.

> Central to the strategy is a new approach to tackling problem drug use based firmly on the concept of recovery. Recovery is a process through which an individual is enabled to move-on from their problem drug use towards a drug-free life and become an active and contributing member of society. Moving to an approach that is based on recovery will mean a significant change in both the pattern of services that are commissioned and in the way that practitioners engage with individuals. The strategy sets in train a number of actions to turn recovery into a reality. Core to this is the reform of the way that drug services are planned, commissioned and delivered to place a stronger emphasis on outcomes and on recovery.
>
> The Government does, however, believe that preventing drug use is more effective than treating established problems. We are taking a broad approach to reducing the future demand for drugs recognising explicitly the strong links between tackling problem drug use and the Government's wider policies such as mental health, early years and growing the economy. This broad approach is complemented by action to improve drugs education, in and outwith, the school environment. We will also continue to provide accurate and credible information on drugs to help reduce recreational drug use.

Reducing the supply of drugs is a vital part of the strategy in order to reduce the harms to individuals and society and protect communities. We are supporting the efforts of the Scottish Crime and Drug Enforcement Agency (SCDEA) to understand better the complex relationship between supply, availability and price of illegal commodities. We are also looking at strengthening further the powers available under the Proceeds of Crime Act 2002 so that a lifetime of crime is open to a lifetime of recovery, and more assets gained through drug dealing can be recycled back to local communities; we are piloting the extension of Drug Treatment and Testing Orders to lower tariff offenders; and improving treatment within prisons.

Finally, the strategy sets out the Government's renewed approach to developing more effective responses to children at risk of parental substance misuse. It sets in motion a programme of action to ensure that the child is at the centre of agency responses and that the principle of early intervention is embedded.

(Scottish Government 2008, pp.vi–vii)

A combined drug and alcohol strategy for Wales was published in 1996. This was primarily intended to address both prevention of the misuse of alcohol and illicit drugs and to provide treatment, support, and rehabilitation of those in need of such assistance (Welsh Office 1996). Since devolution, the joint consideration of alcohol and other drugs in Wales has been consolidated by the Welsh Assembly. This approach has been set out with the following four aims:

to help children, young people and adults resist substance misuse in order to achieve their full potential in society, and to promote sensible drinking in the context of a healthy lifestyle.

to protect families and communities from anti-social behaviour and health risks related to substance misuse.

to enable people with substance misuse problems to overcome them and live healthy and fulfilling lives and in the case of offenders, crime-free lives.

to stifle the availability of illegal drugs on our streets and inappropriate availability of other substances.

(Welsh Office 1996)

A new policy document, *Working Together to Reduce Harm*, was published in 2008 (Welsh Assembly Government 2008). Introducing this 10-year strategy, Dr Brian Gibbons, Minister for Social Justice and Local Government, stated:

The strategy aims to educate and prevent substance misuse, improve services for substance misusers, support and protect families and tackle the availability of illicit drugs and the inappropriate availability of alcohol. The strategy addresses all types of substances, including illegal drugs, over the counter medicines, prescription only medicines and volatile substances such as glue and aerosols but places greatest emphasis on the problems caused by the inappropriate or risky use of alcohol.

(Welsh Assembly Government, press release, 1 October 2008)

A 5-year *Drug Strategy for Northern Ireland* was published in 1999. This focused on four priority areas: young people, communities, treatment and availability (Northern Ireland Office 1999). This has been augmented by the Strategy for Reducing Alcohol Related Harm (Department of Health, Social Services & Public Safety 2000), and the corresponding Model for the Joint Implementation of the Drug & Alcohol Strategies (Department of Health, Social Services & Public Safety 2001). The original strategy has been super-ceded by the New Strategic Direction for Alcohol and Drugs (2006–11) (Department of Health, Social Services & Public Safety 2006). The overall aim of this strategy is to reduce the level of alcohol and drug related harm in Northern Ireland. Its seven specific long term objectives are as follows:

> Provide accessible and effective treatment and support for people who are consuming alcohol and/or using drugs in a potentially hazardous, harmful or dependent way.
>
> Reduce the level, breadth and depth of alcohol and drug-related harm to users, their families and/or their carers and the wider community.
>
> Increase awareness on all aspects of alcohol and drug-related harm in all settings and for all age groups.
>
> Integrate those policies which contribute to the reduction of alcohol and drug related harm into all Government Department strategies.
>
> Develop a competent skilled workforce across all sectors that can respond to the complexities of alcohol and drug use and misuse.
>
> Promote opportunities for those under the age of 18 years to develop appropriate skills, attitudes and behaviours to enable them to resist societal pressures to drink alcohol and/or use illicit drugs, with a particular emphasis on those identified as potentially vulnerable.
>
> Reduce the availability of illicit drugs in Northern Ireland.
>
> (Department of Health, Social Services & Public Safety 2006, p.2)

Chapter 6

The law and the criminal justice system

Marijuana is the most violence-causing drug in the history of mankind.
(Harry Anslinger, US Representative to the United Nations Narcotics Commission 1962)

The links between drug use and crime are clearly established. In fact, around three-quarters of crack and heroin users claim they commit crime to feed their habit.
(Home Office Online 2008a)

It isn't all drug users who commit 'acquisitive' crime such as burglary. In fact, it is only a very small percentage of those who have tried drugs who are also involved in acquisitive crime. Those who are most likely to commit such crimes are people who are dependent on heroin, other opiates or crack cocaine (not cocaine powder), and it's also true that even people addicted to these drugs don't always turn to crime to support their habit.
(DrugScope 2010b)

This chapter summarizes the main provisions of the UK's Misuse of Drugs Act (1971) and other legislation related to illicit drug use. It should be noted that this important piece of legislation is derived from the International United National Convention 1961. This Convention sets out the framework for domestic legislation in member countries but often results in slightly different laws with varying penalties and constraints. For this reason differences are often observed between countries when comparisons are made. It also considers some of the recent debates about the operation of the criminal justice system in relation to drugs and drug users. The legal classification of drugs will be critically considered in the light of evidence suggesting that some legal drugs (such as alcohol and tobacco) are at least as dangerous as some of those which are illegal. A review will also be provided of trends in cautions and convictions for drug-related offences. The overall role of drugs in relation to crime and the criminal justice system will also be considered. This discussion will include the issues of drug offenders, drug dependents and drug use in prison, the impact of drugs on the court service, probation, and Customs and Excise.

Drugs and crime

Illicit drug use, by its very definition, sets the user against the law and makes him or her vulnerable to prosecution. There is no doubt that drug use imposes a massive burden upon the apparatus of law enforcement and the criminal justice system. The situation has been succinctly summarized in the following words:

> At least 1 in 8 arrestees (equivalent to about 125,000 people in England and Wales) are estimated to be problem heroin and/or crack users, compared with about 1 in 100 of the general population.
>
> 81% of arrestees who used heroin and/or crack at least once a week said they committed an acquisitive crime in the previous 12 months, compared with 30% of other arrestees.
>
> 31% reported an average of at least one crime a day, compared with 3% of other arrestees.
>
> Between a third and a half of new receptions to prison are estimated to be problem drug users (equivalent to between 45,000 and 65,000 prisoners in England and Wales).
>
> Drug-related crime costs an estimated £13.5 billion in England and Wales alone.
>
> Problem drug users are much more likely to be found within the criminal justice system (CJS) than within the wider population. There is also strong evidence that problematic use of some drugs, notably heroin and crack, can amplify offending behaviour, and there is a particularly strong association with acquisitive crime, such as shoplifting and burglary. However, for most offenders who use drugs, whose drug use is less extensive, there is no direct causal link between drugs and crime. For example, most are not committing crimes to pay for their drugs.
>
> Problem drug-using offenders have particularly high rates of offending, but they also have high rates of a range of other problems, such as homelessness, unemployment, low educational attainment and disrupted family background, which make the relationship between drugs and crime more complex and the task of rehabilitation more challenging.
>
> (UK Drug Policy Commission 2008, p.7–8)

There are several relevant pieces of legislation in the UK which govern the use and misuse of drugs which are considered to be harmful. Drugs coming into this category are controlled by statute and are monitored by the legal and criminal justice system. The most important acts in the UK are the Misuse of Drugs Act (1971) and the Misuse of Drugs Regulations (1985, updated 2001). The former prohibits certain activities in relation to 'controlled drugs' relating to their manufacture, supply, and possession. These drugs are defined in three classes according to the degree of harm with which they are associated (see below).

The Misuse of Drugs Regulations are concerned with supply and possession of controlled drugs and lay down the conditions under which these activities can be carried out. There are five schedules each specifying the requirements governing activities such as import, export, production, supply, possession, prescribing, and record keeping. Schedule 1 applies to drugs such as LSD and cannabis which have no medical indication. Schedule 2 includes drugs such as heroin, morphine, pethidine, amphetamine, methadone, cocaine, oxycodone, and others. These drugs are controlled under the fullest regulations relating to prescribing, record keeping, and possession. Schedule 3 includes the barbiturates, buprenorphine, mazindol, meprobamate, midazolam, pentazocine, phentermine, and temazepam. They are subject to special prescription requirement (except temazepam) and other restrictions. Schedule 4 includes most of the benzodiazepines and steroids and some hormone preparations. Controls are minimal and prescribing restrictions do not apply. Schedule 5 includes some drugs which appear in other schedules but are in reduced strength. They are not subject to control regulations except the requirement to retain invoices for 2 years (British Medical Association and Royal Pharmaceutical Society of Great Britain 2009).

International conventions, treaties, and regulations also play an important role in the control and distribution of drugs of medical and misuse potential. The International Narcotics Control Board (INCB) is the independent and quasi-judicial monitoring body for the implementation of the United Nations international drug-control conventions. It was established in 1968 in accordance with the Single Convention on Narcotic Drugs, 1961. It had predecessors under the former drug control treaties as far back as the time of the League of Nations. The functions of INCB are laid down in the following treaties: the Single Convention on Narcotic Drugs (1961), the Convention on Psychotropic Substances (1971), and the United Nations Convention Against Illicit Traffic in Narcotic Drugs and Psychotropic Substances (1988).

Drugs and the law

The introduction of the Arsenic Act (1851) and the Poisons Act (1858) were noted in Chapter 1. These were not so much concerned with either drug dependence or the use of drugs for recreational purposes as with their use to poison people. The UK was widely condemned for its opium trading in China. Its policies were reversed as the result of international criticism and international agreements to control drug supplies. The UK was a signatory to the world's first international drug control treaty, the First International Opium Convention of 1912. The Convention was adopted in 1915 by the USA and four other countries: China, Honduras, the Netherlands, and Norway. It became global in 1919 when it was incorporated into the Treaty of Versailles. There were two opium conferences in 1924 and 1925. These were accompanied by the Second Opium Convention of 1924. A modified version of the International Opium Convention was ratified in 1925. This took effect from 1928. The latter was incorporated into UK law under the Coca Leaves and Indian Hemp Regulations of 1928. This legislation included cannabis. Use of the latter was only permitted for medical or scientific purposes. The Opium Convention was eventually superseded by the Single Convention of 1961. The latter has been described in the following terms:

> The adoption of this Convention is regarded as a milestone in the history of international drug control. The Single Convention codified all existing multilateral treaties on drug control and extended the existing control systems to include the cultivation of plants that were grown as the raw material of narcotic drugs. The principal objectives of the Convention are to limit the possession, use, trade in, distribution, import, export, manufacture and production of drugs exclusively to medical and scientific purposes and to address drug trafficking through international cooperation to deter and discourage drug traffickers. The Convention also established the International Narcotics Control Board, merging the Permanent Central Board and the Drug Supervisory Board.
>
> (International Narcotics Control Board 2008b, p.1)

As noted in Chapter 1, cocaine trafficking was identified as a problem in London during the First World War. Measures to restrict this trade were included in the Defence of the Realm Act (1916). This legislation was strengthened in 1917 and reinforced even more by the Dangerous Drugs Act (1920). Nevertheless, abuse of cocaine continued to be problem in London for some years, as is shown by the fact that in 1921, the first year of operation of the Dangerous Drugs Act (1920), out of 67 prosecutions in respect of drugs other than opium, 58 related to cocaine, and in 1922 and 1923 the corresponding figures were 70 out of a total of 110 and 68 out of a total of 128 prosecutions (Jeffery in Phillipson 1970, p.60).

Between the world wars it was reported that the recreational use of illicit drugs declined, although some opium dealing was reported. Alcohol consumption was also low.

During 1924 the Rolleston Committee was convened to assess the British approach to drug use. The Committee produced its report in 1926 and, in so doing, established what has been called the 'British System' of dealing with drug dependence (Schur 1966). Essentially, the Committee interpreted current UK drugs laws to imply that people who were drug-dependent were sick. Moreover, such individuals could be provided with legal supplies of drugs if this helped them to lead 'normal' lives. Doctors who abused this system were to lose their freedom to prescribe drugs. This system worked without much controversy for 20 years. During this period doctors prescribed drugs to a few hundred so-called therapeutic addicts. These were mostly middle-aged people who had become dependent on drugs such as morphine during medical treatment or who had access to such substances through their work. The latter included doctors and nurses. This was a small and stable group of people, most of whom lived 'conventional' lives. The numbers of such individuals who were recorded by the Home Office fell from 700 to fewer than 400 between 1935 and 1955. As noted in Chapter 1, evidence of rising heroin use and dependence was produced by the second Brain Committee report of 1965. The upsurge in drug use in towns and cities throughout Britain prompted journalistic, academic, clinical, and political interest (see Bestic 1966, Bewley. 1966, Dawtry 1968, Kosviner et al. 1968, De Alarcon and Rathod 1968, De Alarcon 1969, Phillipson 1970, Wiener 1970).

The Misuse of Drugs Act (1971)

This is the main piece of legislation covering the control of illicit drugs in the UK. It classifies drugs into three categories, A, B, and C. The Act has been modified since its introduction, mainly to incorporate new substances, such as ecstasy (MDMA), ketamine, mephedrone, and gammahydroxybutrate (GHB or liquid ecstasy) and gammabutyrolactone (GBL). The act was also modified to reclassify cannabis from Class B to Class C in 2004, but this was reversed in January 2009 to return the drug to Class B (see Chapter 8). The Drugs Act (2005) classified raw magic mushrooms as being in Category A.

The Misuse of Drugs Act refers to the drugs that it covers as controlled substances. Class A drugs (such as heroin, crack, and cocaine) are those considered to be the most harmful.

Offences under the Act

Offences under the Act include:

- possession of a controlled substance unlawfully;
- possession of a controlled substance with intent to supply it;
- supplying or offering to supply a controlled drug (even where no charge is made for the drug);
- allowing premises you occupy or manage to be used unlawfully for the purpose of producing or supplying controlled drugs.

Drug trafficking (supply) attracts serious punishment, including life imprisonment, for Class A offences. To enforce this law the police have special powers to stop, detain, and search people on 'reasonable suspicion' that they are in possession of a controlled drug.

Classification under the Act

The ABC classification system is devised to allow the allocation of penalties for possession and dealing these drugs. Drugs are graded according to the harmfulness attributed to a drug when it is misused.

Class A drugs include ecstasy (methylenedioxymethamphetamine, MDMA), lysergide (LSD), diamorphine (heroin), cocaine, crack cocaine, magic mushrooms, amphetamines (if prepared for injection), alfentanil, dipipanone, methadone, morphine, opium, pethidine, phencyclidine (PCP, angel dust), remefentanil, and all class B substances when they are prepared for injection. The penalties for possession are up to 7 years in prison or an unlimited fine, or both. Penalties for dealing are up to life in prison or an unlimited fine, or both.

Class B drugs include oral amphetamines, barbiturates, methylphenidate (ritalin), cannabis, cannabis resin, codeine, ethylmorphine, glutethamide, pentazocine, phenmetrazine, and pholcodine. The penalties for possession are up to 5 years in prison or an unlimited fine, or both. Penalties for dealing are up to 14 years in prison or an unlimited fine, or both.

Class C drugs include some amphetamine-related drugs such as benzfetamine and chlorphentermine, buprenorphine, diethylproprion, mazindol, meprobamate, pemoline, pipradol, most of the benzodiazepines, zolpidem, androgenic and anabolic steroids, gammahydroxybutyrate (GHB), ketamine, clenbuterol, human chorionic gonadotrophin (HCG), non-human chorionic gonadotrophin, somatotrophin, somatrem, and somatropin. The penalties for possession are up to 2 years in prison or an unlimited fine, or both. The penalties for dealing are up to 14 years in prison or an unlimited fine, or both (Home Office Online 2008b).

There is a further division for prescribing purposes. Drugs are allocated into five Schedules under the Misuse of Drugs Regulations 2001 (which is part of the Misuse of Drugs Act 1971) to allow control and restrictions to be placed on prescribing by doctors and nurses.

The Drugs Act (2005)

The 2005 Drugs Act was brought in with the express aim of increasing the powers of the police and the courts. The aims of the Drugs Act were to:

increase the effectiveness of the Drug Interventions Programme by getting more offenders into treatment;

introduce a new civil order that would run alongside anti-social behaviour orders for adults to tackle drug related anti-social behaviour;

enhance police and court powers against drug offenders;

clarify existing legislation in respect of magic mushrooms.

The content of the Drugs Act (2005) is as follows (DrugScope 2010c):

test drug offenders on arrest, rather than on charge;

require a person with a positive test to undergo an assessment by a drugs worker;

provide for an intervention order to be attached to ASBOs issued to adults whose anti-social behaviour is drug related, requiring them to attend drug counselling;

allow a court to remand in police custody for up to a further 192 hours those who swallow drugs in secure packages, to increase the likelihood of the evidence being recovered;

allow a court or jury to draw adverse inference where a person refuses without good cause to consent to an intimate body search, X-ray, or ultrasound scan;

create a new presumption of intent to supply where a defendant is found to be in possession of a certain quantity of controlled drugs;

require courts to take account of aggravating factors—such as dealing near a school—when sentencing;

amend the Anti-Social Behaviour Act (2003) to give police the power to enter premises, such as a crack house, to issue a closure notice;

amend the Misuse of Drugs Act (1971), making fungi containing the drugs psilocin or psilocybin (magic mushrooms) Class A drugs.

A critique of the way in which UK problem drug offenders are managed was produced in March 2008 by the UK Drug Policy Commission (2008). It should be noted that, due to their illegality, a number of aspects of drug use are not easy to investigate. Very little is known about some topics. This situation has been ably summarized (in another context) thus:

> Now what is the message there? The message is that there are known "knowns." There are things we know that we know. There are known unknowns. That is to say there are things that we now know we don't know. But there are also unknown unknowns. There are things we don't know we don't know. So when we do the best we can and we pull all this information together, and we then say well that's basically what we see as the situation, that is really only the known knowns and the known unknowns. And each year, we discover a few more of those unknown unknowns.

> (Donald Rumsfeld 2002)

Because certain types of drug use and related activities (such as producing and supplying drugs) are illicit, less is known about these than about comparable factors connected with, for example, alcohol and tobacco use. One area where evidence is inevitably only partial relates to drug trafficking. Much is known about this, but it is not clear, for example, what volume of illicit drugs is produced and traded. 'Official agencies' such as the police and customs and the military do a huge amount of work attempting to monitor and intercept illicit drug supplies. In spite of this, unknown (but probably huge) quantities evade detection. In addition, as noted in Chapter 3, surveys of self-reported drug use are beset by non-response, under-reporting, and exaggeration.

The UK Drug Policy Commission produced a report entitled *Tackling Drug Markets and Distribution Networks in the UK* (McSweeney et al. 2008). This is an excellent and informative review subject to the problems just noted. The authors of this report conclude that:

> In 2003/04 the size of the UK illicit drug market was estimated to be £5.3 billion. Drug trafficking is considered to be the most profitable sector of transnational criminality and to pose the single greatest organised crime threat to the UK. The size of the UK market means it is extremely lucrative for drug traffickers–both in scale and in terms of the profits that can be made. Estimated lifetime prevalence of cannabis use–globally the most widely consumed illicit drug–is higher in England and Wales than in any other European country. The UK also has a higher proportion of problem drug users within the adult population than any of its European neighbours. The illicit drugs trade in the UK has far-reaching political, cultural and economic ramifications, and impacts negatively upon prison populations, levels of gun crime, social exclusion, and public health and community safety. These consequences and impacts are experienced disproportionately by the urban poor and minority ethnic groups.

> (McSweeney et al. 2008, pp.7–8)

The report provides a detailed overview of what is known about the UK drug market. The authors note that UK drug expenditure is distributed as follows: crack cocaine 28%, heroin 23%, cannabis 20%, cocaine 18%, amphetamines 6%, and ecstasy 5%. The drug market (on the basis of what is known about it) has been estimated by Pudney et al. (2006) as being equivalent to approximately 33% and 41% respectively of the UK alcohol and tobacco markets (McSweeney et al. 2008).

Drug offences

In addition to drug offences recorded within the UK, the UK Foreign and Commonwealth Office has reported that such crimes top the list of why British citizens are arrested and convicted overseas. A disproportionate number of such offences are committed in Spain. In addition, some Britons are convicted of drugs offences in countries, such as Thailand, where the death penalty is imposed for drug trafficking. It was reported in early 2010 that 1000 British citizens were convicted of drug offences in other countries (BBC News Online, 3 February, 2010a). It had been previously noted that 22 British citizens had recently been sentenced to death for drugs offences in countries such as China, Thailand, Malaysia, and Singapore (Sky News 2009).

Drugs in prison

UK prisons have long been increasingly severely overcrowded and in a state of crisis. The UK has the highest rate of incarceration in Western Europe. At the time of writing over 90 000 men and women are locked up in UK prisons. Many of these individuals have mental health problems and/or alcohol and drug-related problems. The impact of drugs on the prison system is massive. Cannabis has replaced tobacco as a commonplace type of prison currency and it is easy to obtain a variety of drugs in prison. Many prisoners use drugs and a substantial proportion are believed to drug-dependent (Farrell et al. 2002). A study of the treatment needs of sentenced male prisoners with psychiatric disorders indicated that 8.6% were alcohol-dependent and 10.1% were drug-dependent (Gunn et al. 1991). A more recent picture of the very serious levels of psychiatric disorders (including alcohol and drug dependence) among men and women in the prison population has been given by Singleton et al. (1998). This is summarized by Table 6.1.

Gunn et al. (1991) found that 10.1% of prisoners were drug-dependent. Maden et al. (1990, 1992) found that 23% of female prison inmates and 11% of males were dependent on drugs during the 6 months before they were incarcerated. A more recent study Singleton et al. (1998) indicated that 34% were drug-dependent. A prison survey in England and Wales indicated that over 60% of heroin and cannabis users had taken drugs in prison. More than 25% of the heroin users had begun to use this drug while in prison (Boys et al. 2002). May (2005) has reported that the drugs most commonly taken by offenders in the 30 days prior to custody are heroin (62%), crack cocaine (49%),

Table 6.1 The prevalence of psychiatric disorders among sentenced and remand prisoners in England and Wales (%)

Disorder/condition	Sentenced men	Sentenced women	Remand men	Remand women
Schizophrenic or delusional disorder	6	13	9	13
Affective psychosis	1	2	2	2
Neurotic disorder	40	63	59	76
Personality disorder	64	50	78	50
Alcohol dependence	30	19	30	20
Drug dependence	34	36	43	52
Suicide attempt*	7	16	15	27
Self-harm in prison	7	10	5	9

*In the past year.

(*Source*: UK Statistics Authority website: www.statisticsauthority.gov.uk or ww.statistics.gov.uk. Crown Copyright material is reproduced with the permission of the Controller, Office of Public Sector Information (OPSI). Adapted from Singleton et al. 1998)

and cannabis (42%). May also notes that the drug most often identified as the main problem substance by inmates assessed by the CARAT drug service in prisons was heroin. Prisoners also reported that the average amount spent on drugs each week prior to imprisonment was £590. Those spending the most were women (£810) and those whose main offences were theft/handling, robbery, and burglary (£670).

Former military personnel

It has long been evident that many of the men and women who have served in the military develop problems with legal or illicit drugs. One of the classic studies of drug use is Lee Robins' celebrated longitudinal investigation of the progress of opiate-using Vietnam veterans after returning to the USA (Robins 1973, 1974). This showed that the majority ceased to use heroin after completing their military service. Returning to her cases at a later stage Robins was able to show that a significant number of these individuals had relapsed into heroin use after returning home (Robins et al. 1980).

Some ex-service personnel are not so fortunate. Many suffer from post-traumatic stress disorder (PTSD) and depression, together with alcohol and drug problems. The recent conflicts in Northern Ireland, Bosnia, Iraq, and Afghanistan appear to have increased the emotional pressures on those serving in these areas. It was reported in September 2009 that 20 000 former military personnel were currently in the UK's criminal justice system (Travis 2009b). This suggested that a far higher proportion of the imprisoned population were ex-military personnel than the 4%–6% previously suggested by Home Office research (Crawford 2008).

> The proportion of veterans in the prison population has more than doubled in six years, according to a report published today highlighting the hidden cost of recent military action.
>
> About 12,000 veterans are on probation or parole, representing 6 per cent of the total, while 8,500 are in prison, representing 8.5 per cent of the jail population, according to the report by the National Association of Probation Officers (Napo).
>
> The figures suggest that more ex-servicemen and women are in the criminal justice system of England and Wales than there are troops serving in Afghanistan.
>
> Misuse of alcohol and drugs are key factors behind offending by veterans and a high proportion of crimes are linked to domestic violence. The association said that the Services should do more to tackle alcohol misuse as well as provide programmes to deal with domestic violence.
>
> (Ford 2009, p.1)

Contemporary discussion on drug and alcohol control and legislation

There is always an ongoing series of drug and alcohol issues which are top of the agenda of concern for politicians. At the present time there is a need to address the acute problems of excessive alcohol use by young people. The need for legislation is recognized by many academics and politicians and is supported by at least a section of the public. The interaction between the medical profession and politics was demonstrated when Sir Liam Donaldson, Chief Medial Officer for England, called for a minimum unit price of 50 pence to be introduced.

This recommendation was based upon evidence that such a step would particularly affect harmful and hazardous drinkers. It would also reduce alcohol-related mortality by over 3000 deaths per year as well as cutting hospital admissions by 97 900 per year, crimes by 45 800 per year, and sickness leave by 296 900 days per year. This step, it was calculated, would also reduce the cost associated with such problems by £1 billion annually (Meier et al. 2008). Sir Liam's recommendation was peremptorily rejected by Prime Minister Gordon Brown even before it was officially made public by Sir Liam. Brown stated that:

> We do not want the responsible, sensible majority of moderate drinkers to have to pay more or suffer as a result of the excesses of a small minority. And that's the context in which we look at the problems that the chief medical officer has raised.
>
> (Hencke and Sparrow 2009)

The Prime Minister's response was in keeping with the policy of successive Labour and Conservative governments in relation to alcohol. Repeated scientific and medical pleas to the government (including by its own advisors) to save many thousands of lives and substantially reduce alcohol problems by using taxation have for decades been rejected. During November 2009 the Scottish Government published proposals to reduce Scotland's chronic alcohol problems (Scottish Government 2008). These included the recommendation that a minimum unit price should be introduced. This approach, supported by a review of taxation options and discount bans in Scotland (Meier et al. 2009), was given strong and enthusiastic backing from medical and scientific authorities. In spite of this the other main political parties at Holyrood (Conservative, Labour, and Liberal Democrat) opposed these measures, justifying this with some rather peculiar explanations. These included the claim that minimum unit pricing would not affect the consumption of Buckfast tonic wine! One of the authors discussed this with several MSPs whose opposition appeared to be at least partly attributable to dislike of the Scottish National Party, the current administration at Holyrood.

Scientific and medical advice has been met with open disdain. Instead political parties and governments (urged on by the powerful alcoholic beverage industry) have opted for notoriously ineffective approaches, including media campaigns and alcohol education (Plant and Plant 2006). The arguments over scientific advice in general and drug classification in particular will probably continue to rumble on. At the time of writing it appears possible that drug control laws may be extended to apply to substances or mixtures of substances that are currently 'legal drugs'. These include 'herbal ecstasy,' yohimbine or 'herbal viagra,' 'spice' (herbs with some cannabis-like effects), and 'herbal ecstasy' (benzylpiperazine, BZP; a stimulant with amphetamine-like effects) (Holford and Cass 2002, Gottlieb 2006, Doward and Shah 2009). During July 2009 the Advisory Council on the Misuse of Drugs (ACMD) produced a report on the synthetic cannabinoid receptor agonists (cannabinoid agonists or synthetic cannabinoids). The latter includes the smoking mixture called spice (Advisory Committee on the Misuse of Drugs 2009b). The ACMD called upon the Government to ban Spice Gold, a popular smoking mixture:

> Spice Gold, and other types of blend that offer users a similar sensation to cannabis, is dangerous, according to the government's Advisory Council on the Misuse of Drugs (ACMD).
>
> "These are not harmless herbal alternatives and have been found to cause paranoia and panic attacks," said ACMD Chairman Professor David Nutt.
>
> The demand for herbal highs in Britain has increased rapidly, with a number of online sites and so-called "head shops" that sell legal drug paraphernalia reporting they have sold out of Spice Gold. Spice Gold is made up of ingredients including dried flowers and leaves but the ACMD says it is coated with synthetic cannabinoids that imitate the effect of the active ingredient in cannabis.

"Young people think they are safer herbal alternatives to cannabis but they have the potential to be more harmful because users don't know the mixture and quantity of chemicals in the product," it warned.

An average 3-gram bag costs between 20-25 pounds and smokers can choose from flavours such as 'diamond', 'tropical' and 'Arctic.'

The mixture, which is said to smell like honey, marshmallow and vanilla, is already banned in many European countries including Germany and Austria.

Ulrich Zimmermann from Dresden Technical University, who published a report on the withdrawal effects of Spice Gold in July, said it was more dangerous than cannabis.

"People don't actually know what the ingredients are – nobody knows what people add into those herbal blends. Nobody knows whether they are safe," he said.

(Master 2009, p.1)

It should be noted that an earlier report on spice had been produced by the European Monitoring Centre for Drugs and Drug Addiction (EMCDDA 2009b). This also concluded that this drug had dangerous effects. It also noted that it appeared to be in use in several European countries, although the extent of such use was unclear. The ACMD's recommendation to control some of the existing 'legal highs,' such as cannabinoids, was supported by the charity DrugScope. Even so, the latter also called for a thorough review of the system of drug classification:

In light of recent decisions by the Government not to follow the ACMD's advice on cannabis and ecstasy classification and the need to respond appropriately and proportionately to new substances and harms, it is time that the classification system was reviewed. Such a review was promised by the Government in January 2006 and subsequently abandoned.

(DrugScope 2009c, p.1)

During August 2009 the Home Office announced that herbal ecstasy (BZP) and another legal high known as GBL, together with the cannabinoids noted above, would be banned before the end of the year. The cannabis-like drugs would be classified as Category B drugs, while GBL (originally used as an industrial solvent) and BZP would be classified as Category C drugs. It was noted that herbal ecstasy had recently been linked with small number of deaths. Both BZP and GBL were associated with 'heart problems, vomiting, anxiety attacks, mood swings and seizures' (BBC News Online, 25 August, 2009d). Another drug that has been causing concern is called mephodrone, sometimes known as legal cocaine, drone, or bubble, a legal high that is becoming widely used as a dance drug. It has been reported that use by teenagers is increasing and that some have sought medical help related to their use. Mephodrone is reputed to cause effects that are similar to those obtained from using ecstasy: euphoria, alertness, sociability, and feelings of empathy. The reported adverse effects of this drug include 'nose bleeds, and burns, paranoia, heart palpitations, insomnia and memory problems'. Some users have had to be resuscitated after their hearts stopped beating. It has also been reported to foster aggression (Campbell 2010). The ACMD has been reported as likely to recommend that mephodrone should be classified under the Misuse of Drugs Act.

A range of herbal highs were banned in December 2009. It was widely reported that this step was at least partly prompted by the death of medical student Hester Stewart 8 months previously. She had reportedly taken a mixture of alcohol and GBL prior to her demise. GBL was classified as a Category C drug under the Misuse of Drugs Act. It was noted that the latest drug to cause concern was mephodrone. Home Office sources reported that research into the effects of this drug was required urgently as a preliminary to the possible control of the drug.

Drugs in the future

As earlier chapters have indicated, a lot is known about drugs and drug use. Even so, our evidence is neither complete nor flawless. An ambitious exercise in predicting the future was undertaken by Foresight, an impressive group whose key scientific advisors included Professors David Nutt, Trevor Robbins, and Gerry Stimson. This initiative was commissioned by the Office of Science and Technology. The Foresight brief was to consider 'How can we manage the use of psychoactive substances in the future to best advantage for the individual, the community and society?' It involved discussions (of a very mixed quality) involving disparate, multidisciplinary groups of people involved in the drug field. The resulting report, entitled *Drug Futures* was released in 2007 (Foresight 2007). Its conclusions included the following:

> There have been significant advances in our understanding of addiction and our understanding of the treatments available for it.
>
> The amount of information on the harms of 'recreational' drugs is increasing.
>
> We may be able to use this growing body of evidence to help us to make better decisions about our 'recreational' use of them. For example, it is clear that children and adolescents are much more vulnerable than adults to harm and addiction.
>
> Drugs are being developed which help people to forget experiences. In the future it might be possible to 'unlearn' an addiction.
>
> Vaccines are being trialled that might allow us to stop the action of specific 'recreational' psychoactive substances on the brain.
>
> Genomics is helping us to identify why certain groups of people are at greater risk of harm from 'recreational' drugs than others. This could allow treatments to be targeted more precisely.
>
> A drug has been found that can block the memory-impairing actions of alcohol in humans.

New types of so-called 'recreational' psychoactive substances are being developed.
Scientists have been able to separate the effect of one psychoactive substance from its addictive properties. This could pave the way to non-addictive 'recreational' drugs, but as with any new substance the risks will need to be assessed also.

A psychoactive substance has been developed that reduces the side-effects of 'recreational' drugs. Such compounds might allow users to shape their drug experience.

Scientists believe that they could produce a 'recreational' substance with similar effects to alcohol but fewer harms.

(Foresight 2007, p.9)

These conclusions were part of a much wider-ranging and futuristic review of possible developments in the drug field. One possibility that attracted media attention was that of the development of 'non-addictive recreational drugs'. In fact this suggestion (reminiscent of synthehol from the television series *Star Trek*; this fictional chemical tastes like alcohol, but lacks its harmful effects) provoked some scepticism and debate. It was pointed out that a number of existing drugs (heroin, amphetamines, and benzodiazepines) had been promoted as being problem-free at some stage before the problems associated with them were fully recognized. Prediction is a bold and uncertain process. Today's science fiction often becomes tomorrow's reality. Even so, science has been making rapid progress in many areas, so at least some of the above possibilities may be realized in time. Another point is that even if non-addictive drugs do become available they may not replace today's harmful substances. Many people like taking risks.

Chapter 7

Does drug education make any difference?

Politicians of all political hues appear seldom able to resist the lure of high-profile, populist responses to illicit drug use and its associated problems. A number of twentieth century anti-drug initiatives and activities involved the promotion of fearsome, shocking images intended to scare people away from drugs. Examples of these included the lurid film *Reefer Madness* (also known as *Tell your Children*) from 1936. This depicted a series of tragic events befalling young people who smoked cannabis. It has subsequently been used for amusement by drug users as well as being turned into a musical. Sometimes popular discussion of drugs and drug issues has been driven not so much by a wish to educate as by a wish to frighten. This has sometimes influenced the nature of what passes for 'drug education'. Initiatives in the UK have sometimes been strongly influenced by the policies and practices of the USA. The latter has driven the War on Drugs as well as some of the ways in which drug education has been approached. During the 1980s the Conservative Government supported the US hard line on drug controls. Margaret Thatcher (and Princess Diana) also endorsed Nancy Reagan's 'just say no' approach to youthful drug use (Schlosser 2004). The subsequent 1980s national AIDS awareness campaign was characterized by grim warnings of death portrayed by dark scenes of tombstones and skeletal young people who were supposed to be heroin injectors. Evaluations reported the educational value to be mainly for the low-risk non-drug-using population.

Drug education and media anti-drug campaigns have featured prominently in the armoury of the public response to drugs, both in the UK and elsewhere. The most widespread and heavily promoted international drug education programme is Drug Abuse Resistance Education, or DARE:

> This year millions of school children around the world will benefit from D.A.R.E. (Drug Abuse Resistance Education), the highly acclaimed program that gives kids the skills they need to avoid involvement in drugs, gangs, and violence. D.A.R.E. was founded in 1983 in Los Angeles and has proven so successful that it is now being implemented in 75 percent of our nation's school districts and in more than 43 countries around the world. D.A.R.E. is a police officer-led series of classroom

lessons that teaches children from kindergarten through 12th grade how to resist peer pressure and live productive drug and violence-free lives.

(www.ci.morganton.nc.us/index.php/departments/public-safety/140-field-operations-bureau)

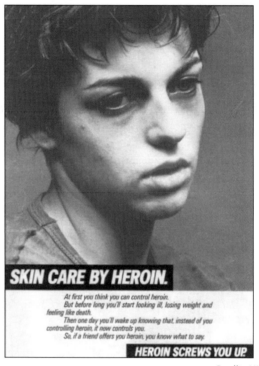

Credit: HM Government.

In fact the actual effectiveness of DARE is controversial. A number of reports cite evidence suggesting that it has not reduced drug use or changed attitudes to drugs:

Does DARE work?

No. All the major research on the effectiveness of DARE shows that it has no impact on the rate of drug use by children who go through DARE training. These reports include:

- ◆ 1991 Kentucky study - National Institute on Drug Abuse - 'No statistically significant differences'
- ◆ 1990 Canadian Government study 'DARE had no significant effect on the use of…marijuana, acid, heroin, crack, glue and PCP'
- ◆ 1993 Research Triangle Institute - National Institute of Justice - Statistical analysis of all DARE research, which says DARE has 'a limited to essentially nonexistent effect' on drug use.

♦ The final edition of the largest evaluation of the DARE program has concluded that the Anti-Drug program does not reduce drug use, and in at least category of pot, the DARE graduates smoked more frequently than the control. The report concluded: 'The DARE program's limited effect on adolescent drug use contrasts with the program's popularity and prevalence. An important implication is that DARE could be taking the place of other, more beneficial drug education programs that kids could be receiving'.

Among the notable quotations from researchers: 'It is well established that DARE doesn't work' Gilbert Botvin - Cornell Medical Center. 'Research shows that, no, DARE hasn't been effective in reducing drug use' William Modzeleski, Top Drug education official at the Department of Education'.

(www.druglibrary.org/schaffer/library/daremenu.htm)

'In 1994 DARE invaded the serenity of our home', Steve Finichel, a doctor from New Jersey told us last fall. 'My 10 year old son began to cry uncontrollably at dinner, informing his mother and me that the wine we were about to drink takes 14 minutes from our lives. He also informed us that we were alcoholics. To make matters worse, he put a tip into the classroom DARE box and was frightened that soon we would be taken off to jail'.

(Eyle 2001–2002, p.1).

A recent review by the US General Accounting Office examined six separate evaluations of DARE. This review followed students for up to a decade after their participation in the programme at 10–11 years of age. Findings again indicated that the programme did not change students' drug-related knowledge, attitudes, or resistance to peer pressure (Vastag 2003). In fact DARE, for all its star support, publicity, and hype, was classified as an 'ineffective program' in 2001 by the US Surgeon General. It would clearly be a major cause for rejoicing if educating young (or older) people about illicit drugs led them to avoid such substances or to avoid the associated risks. A huge amount of money has been spent on drug education in some countries, notably the USA. In the case of the UK, while the total drug education budget is unclear, it is known that some media anti-drugs campaigns have been expensive:

A big boost in backing for Scotland's national anti-drugs campaign was announced today by Deputy Justice Minister Iain Gray at a drugs summit with First Minister Henry McLeish, Cabinet Office Minister Ian McCartney and UK Anti-Drugs Co-ordinator Keith Hellawell.

Scotland Against Drugs (SAD) has been awarded a 50 per cent increase in core funding by the Scottish Executive to £4.5 million over the next three years. This is the first in a series of announcements by Ministers over coming weeks designed to free Scotland from the drugs scourge.

(Scottish Government 2001)

The UK Government's 1998 and 2008 Drug Strategies have given drug education an important role. The 2008 strategy notes the following:

> Young people need credible, balanced information about the risks posed by drugs, which complements drug education delivered in school and other settings. Parents need information to build knowledge, to provide reassurance and to develop the confidence to address drug use issues within the family. Communication also plays a key role in the community, providing reassurance and strengthening confidence and resilience, where communities are aware of the action that is being taken to tackle drug dealing and drug-related crime. Our knowledge of what works in communications has developed substantially since the publication of the 1998 strategy. We are now offering credible and well used drug advice and information, using the kinds of media most used by the target audience, including the internet, magazines and social networking sites. As an example FRANK has become established as a widely recognised and trusted helpline website, and its advertising and related activity has brought about a shift in young people's attitudes to drugs, with more perceiving drugs negatively. Following FRANK multi-media cannabis campaign, research showed there was a 12 per cent increase in the number of young people agreeing with the statement that 'cannabis can damage the mind of someone who uses it', and 89 per cent reported that they knew about FRANK and what its purpose was.
>
> (HM Government 2008a, p.33)

More depressing evidence of the poor performance of drug education appeared during December 2009:

> In the British context, it was expected to decide whether an evidence-based, well structured and well resourced drug education programme could contribute to reducing youth substance use, yet the multi-million pound Blueprint study never got near fulfilling its promise. Though nothing definitive could be concluded from the study, signs were that in both knowledge and prevention terms, the lessons were not an advance on routine personal, social and health education.
>
> (Drug and Alcohol Findings 2009)

This report related to the Blueprint Drug Education Programme. This had been piloted in 23 schools in the East Midlands and north-west England.

It should be acknowledged that there is a difference between drug education and anti-drugs campaigns. Many of the latter have been mainly motivated by a wish to deter young people in particular from using drugs by whatever means is thought to be appropriate. Such campaigns may certainly be regarded as being a form of propaganda, while some have little claim to being either educational or evidence-based. Drug education is often inspired by the wish to prevent or discourage people from using drugs. Even so, it is widely assumed that as 'education' it will have at least some factual (and accurate) content. Many people, including drug educators, assume that drug education does deter people from drugs. Some practitioners and other 'stakeholders' are extremely indignant if confronted by the suggestion that they may not be discouraging people from using drugs (e.g. Elliot 1995). Sadly, this conclusion is supported by what is now a huge international literature. The fact that drug (and alcohol) education has a very poor track record has been evident for decades (e.g. Kalb 1975, Milgram 1976, 1987, Kinder et al. 1980, Schaps et al. 1981, Bandy and President 1983, Pickens 1985, Tobler 1986, Gliksman and Smythe 1990, Edwards et al. 1995, Plant et al. 1997, Foxcroft et al. 1997, 2003, Hawthorne 2001, Babor et al. 2003, Canning et al. 2004, Crombie et al. 2005).

Very few programmes appear to have led to reductions in the use of illicit drugs (Canning et al. 2004, Midford and McBride 2004, McBride 2005, Poulin and Nicholson 2005). Most educational programmes do not appear to have changed drug-use behaviour. Worryingly, some even appear to have increased youthful drug use, both illicit and legal (e.g. Hawthorne et al. 1995).

A sobering comment on the disappointing impact of most drug education initiatives has been provided by Gliksman and Smyth (1990):

> The history of successes of school-based drug education programs has not been a positive one. The general consensus appears to be that although there are individual successes, school-based drug education prevention programs, regardless of their underlying principles, have generally not proven themselves to be effective or are inconsistent in their effectiveness at best. Any positive effects from these programs, have been with respect to changes in knowledge. Changes in attitudes are not consistently found and positive changes in behavior are rarely found to be associated with these programs. We are left with the hope that this knowledge gain will ultimately be instrumental in changing attitudes and behavior, an assumption that we cannot make with any degree of certainty (Goodstadt 1989).
>
> However, before we dismiss the benefits of school-based programming out of hand, we should re-examine two possibilities for the negative view espoused above—that problems of methodology and or a lack of integration of approaches may account for a lack of positive findings. Previously, we suggested that poorly designed studies that ask the wrong questions have been the reason for a lack of positive findings, and suggested that this may indeed be a poor excuse. However, the possibility exists that this is indeed an accurate statement. In fact, Milgram (1987), in the course of articulating a variety of potential reasons for the lack of positive findings, suggests that this may in fact happen with regularity. The potential reasons include the following: (i) the goals of the program may be non-specific making outcome assessment difficult; (ii) the program content may not meet student needs; (iii) teachers delivering the program may be untrained and or uncomfortable with the material; (iv) programs may not be lengthy enough to be effective; and (v) evaluations of these programs may not be conceived properly so that the right questions are not asked. Some of these are problems associated with the program and others are problems of evaluation design. While all are possible, it seems unlikely that methodological issues are high on the list of possibilities.

(Gliksman and Smyth 1990, p.180)

It appears that the most likely outcome of drug education is to temporarily increase knowledge or to change attititudes for a short time. This might be worth doing, but it is a long way from the reduced drug use that many people appear to expect. Brown (2001) has noted that drug education is widespread in spite of the lack of evidence of effectiveness. This, he suggests, is at least partly due to the influence of vested interests. A more positive and constructive note has been provided by the National Institute on Drug Abuse (2003):

> Drug information alone, however, has not been found to be effective in deterring drug abuse. Combining information with skills, methods, and services produces more effective results. Programs include skills development training to build and improve behaviours in important areas, such as communication within the family, social and emotional development, academic and social competence in children, and peer resistance strategies in adolescents.
>
> (National Institute on Drug Abuse 2003, p.22)

The good intentions of governments and educational authorities cannot be denied. Neither can the importance of doing something in an attempt to mitigate the serious consequences of young people starting to use drugs and lacking simple information about protecting themselves from harm. For educationalists and policy makers there are many complex issues which frustrate the development of programmes with an ability to influence the choices of young people. Fashion often dictates behaviour and fashion relies and depends on change, innovation, and novelty. As in other areas of human behaviour new trends arrive regularly and without warning and the serious consequences are often unintended. Almost inevitably education and public health are therefore in a position of responding to a crisis or an unexpected problem arising out of a previously unknown side effect of drug use. Numerous examples show how difficult it is to research and implement an appropriate response to an emerging problem and how often, lacking the ability to predict the future, policies seem to be misguided or ineffective.

Chapter 8

Can drug classification and drug policy ever be evidence-based?

We know no spectacle so ridiculous as the British public in one of its periodic fits of morality.
(Lord Macaulay 1830)

The popular and political debate about illicit drugs has been accused of being at least in part a 'moral panic'. This, as noted above, is an expression originally used by the social scientist Stanley Cohen (1972) to describe exaggerated alarm provoked by some form of behaviour that was viewed as being socially unacceptable and menacing. Cohen applied this term to media coverage of conflict between gangs of 'mods' and 'rockers'. The term moral panic has subsequently been used to imply that the debates on some issues are distorted and sensationalized. There are certainly times when popular concerns about some issues, often whipped up by the tabloid press, are exaggerated and appear to lead to moral (or immoral) outrage. During recent decades, sensationalized reports in Britain have related to a series of drug themes. These have included the use of amphetamines, cannabis, (more recently skunk), soft drugs leading to the use of harder drugs, drug dealers allegedly accosting school children, and drug adulteration. This chapter considers two main issues, the classification of drugs and the very important topic of who determines drug policy. The latter topic received enormous publicity while this book was being written.

Drug classification: reclassify all drugs?

There has long been disagreement about what some view as the arbitrary nature of the existing system of drug classification under the Misuse of Drugs Act (1971). A report from the Science and Technology Committee of the House of Commons had reached the following conclusion:

> With respect to the ABC classification system, we have identified significant anomalies in the classification of individual drugs and a regrettable lack of consistency in the rationale used to make classification decisions. In addition, we have expressed concern at the Government's proclivity for using the classification system as a means

of 'sending out signals' to potential users and society at large—it is at odds with the stated objective of classifying drugs on the basis of harm and the Government has not made any attempt to develop an evidence base on which to draw in determining the 'signal' being sent out.

(Science and Technology Committee 2006)

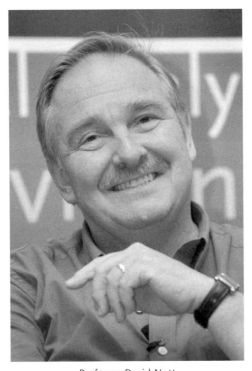

Professor David Nutt
Credit: AP/Press Association Images.

A review by Professor David Nutt (one of those who had given evidence to the above committee) and colleagues concluded that the following would be a more rational classification of overall drug dangers:

1 heroin (most harmful),

2 cocaine,

3 barbiturates,

4 street methadone,

5 alcohol,

6 ketamine,

7 benzodiazepines,

8 amphetamine,

9 tobacco,

10 buprenorphine,

11 cannabis,

12 solvents,

13 4-MTA (*para*-methylthioamphetamine),

14 LSD,

15 methylphenidate (ritalin),

16 anabolic steroids,

17 gammahydroxybutyrate (GHB),

18 ecstasy,

19 alkyl nitrites,

20 khat (least harmful).

(Source: Nutt et al. 2007)

Nutt and his coauthors have noted that this classification (which includes alcohol and tobacco) provides an 'evidence-based' approach, taking account of (1) physical harm to the drug user, (2) the drug's propensity to induce dependence in the user, and (3) the effect of the drug's use on families, communities, and society. Nine assessment parameters were used to devise the classification (which was then considered by two groups of assessors). These were as shown in Table 8.1. This thoughtful, logical, classification certainly appears to a big improvement from both scientific and common-sense perspectives to that

Table 8.1 Nine assessment parameters used to devise the evidence-based classification of Nutt et al

Category	Assessment parameters
Physical harm	Acute
	Chronic
	Intravenous
Dependence	Intensity of pleasure
	Psychological dependence
	Physical dependence
Social harms	Intoxication
	Other social harms
	Health care costs

enshrined in the Misuse of Drugs Act. The fact that alcohol and tobacco, which cause far more harm than illicit drugs, are included by Nutt et al. acknowledges the realities of both their dangers and the extent of the associated damage to both the individual and society at large. The proposal to introduce a 'Misuse of Substances Act' that incorporates alcohol and tobacco along with illicit drugs, has also been recommended by the Commission on Illegal Drugs, Communities and Public Policy of the Royal Society for the Encouragement of Arts, Manufactures and Commerce (2007). Although in many ways a logical approach, the inclusion of alcohol and tobacco, drugs that are legal, with illicit drugs also presents some major problems. The enormous harm associated with these drugs is both obvious and very well documented. Even so, 'society' has long decreed that these addictive and toxic drugs are legal and that they should be treated differently from drugs which are not. Longstanding popular sentiment has turned against tobacco. Smoking is far less socially acceptable than it was several decades ago. This change has facilitated the introduction of stronger measures to curb the use of this drug, such as smoking bans applying to public spaces. Public and political concerns about 'binge drinking'—with its associated public-disorder and other negative effects—-have also prompted measures, such as raising the price of alcoholic beverages (in March 2008) that were formerly politically unacceptable. Even so, the proposition that alcohol and tobacco should be treated exactly as though they were illicit drugs is politically naïve. This review did not attract much attention until late 2009, when it became a political hot potato. It should be noted that many researchers judge it to be factually correct and quite reasonable. A similar review has, for example, been published in France (Roques 1998).

There has periodically been discussion about the current classification of illicit drugs. As noted in Chapter 5, the Police Foundation (2000) recommended reclassifying cannabinnol, LSD, ecstasy, and buprenorphine. This recommendation was not well received either politically or by the popular media. Cannabis has long been the particular focus of a political debate. During the 1970s the Wootton Report on cannabis (Advisory Committee on Drug Dependence 1968) reached the following conclusions:

> An increasing number of people, mainly young, in all classes of society are experimenting with this drug, and substantial numbers use it regularly for social pleasure.
>
> There is no evidence that this activity is causing violent crime or aggression, anti-social behaviour, or is producing in otherwise normal people conditions of dependence or psychosis, requiring medical treatment.
>
> The experience of many other countries is that once it is established cannabis-smoking tends to spread. In some parts of Western society where interest in mood-altering drugs is growing, there are indications that it may become a functional equivalent of alcohol.

In spite of the threat of severe penalties and considerable effort at enforcement the use of cannabis in the United Kingdom does not appear to be diminishing. There is a body of opinion that criticises the present legislative treatment of cannabis on the grounds that it exaggerates the dangers of the drug, and needlessly interferes with civil liberty.

(Advisory Committee on Drug Dependence 1968)

These findings might appear very balanced and reasonable to many contemporary readers. Even so, the report was highly controversial at the time. Some sections of the mass media angrily denigrated the report as 'a junkies' charter'. It was debated in Parliament in a way that suggested that some senior politicians, such as Quentin Hogg and James Callaghan, were at least as concerned to display their moral opposition to drug use in general and to cannabis use in particular, as to consider scientific evidence on drug dangers. Political posturing and indifference to scientific evidence has continued to be a prominent feature of the cannabis debate (Hinscliff 2008). Scientific evidence has often indicated that cannabis is far less dangerous than is sometimes supposed, certainly by politicians.

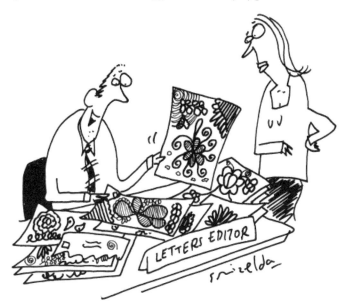

"We've had a lot of post on the legalization of cannabis."

Credit: Cartoon Stock.com.

In 1978 the Advisory Council on the Misuse of Drugs (ACMD) recommended reclassifying cannabis (then in Class B) to Class C. The current Home Secretary,

Merlyn Rees, rejected this suggestion. In March 2002 the ACMD once more recommended that cannabis should be reclassified as a Category C drug. Offences in this category carry lighter penalties than those under Categories A and B. The Home Secretary, David Blunkett, accepted this recommendation. In June 2002 he announced proposals to reclassify cannabis from Class B to Class C. He stressed that reclassification did not imply either decriminalistion or legalization of cannabis. It was also stressed that this change was intended to allow the police to concentrate more effort on Class A drugs such as heroin. Keith Hellawell, then 'drug czar', objected to this change. He resigned his position in July 2002.

As noted in Chapter 6, Class B includes bodybuilding drugs (anabolic steroids), GHB, and some anti-depressants. Cannabis possession would no longer necessarily be an arrestable offence, even though the police would retain discretion to make arrests, for example, if cannabis was smoked near a school. The maximum penalties attached to Category B drugs include 5 years in prison, plus an unlimited fine, for possession and 14 years in prison plus an unlimited fine for supplying/drug dealing and for possession with intent to supply to others. The corresponding maximum penalties associated with possession of Category C drugs are less severe: 2 years in prison plus an unlimited fine for possession. However, the penalties for supply/dealing and for possession with intent to supply others are the same as for Category B drugs.

It appears that there has been considerable confusion about the implications of this change. Some lawyers reported that the reclassification was 'a shambles'. Moreover, Sir John Stevens, Chief Constable for the Metropolitan Police, stated that there was a massive amount of 'muddle' about the new legal status of cannabis. He said that police officers were instructed 'not to arrest adults for using cannabis in their own homes and only to confiscate cannabis if used in public. Even so, anyone using it near schools and all under 18s will still face arrest' (Davenport 2004). It was also evident that the implementation of the new cannabis regulations may not have been uniform throughout the UK. Scottish police were instructed to continue to record all cannabis offences, whereas their colleagues in England were not. Jenkins (2004) even noted that police officers in different parts of London were given different guidelines for enforcing the law related to cannabis. A survey carried out by *The Guardian* in January 2004 confirmed the existence of:

> widespread confusion and inconsistencies about how the police will enforce the new law on cannabis.... Some will operate a strict "arrest all" policy even for possession of small amounts while in other areas, officers will caution adults found with modest amounts, preferring to concentrate their efforts on harder drugs.... In Scotland the deputy Justice Minister Hugh Henry said there would be no change in practice. Although reclassification applies across the UK. Policing and law enforcement are devolved responsibilities.

(Carter 2004)

The Conservative leader at the time, Michael Howard, opposed the reclassification of cannabis and committed any future Conservative government to reversing it (Grice 2004).

The reclassification took effect on 29 January 2004. Thousands of posters and leaflets were circulated to explain this change in schools, colleges, workplaces, and voluntary and community organizations. In addition, large newspaper advertisements were published on that day. These carried the following statement, issued jointly by the Home Office and the Association of Chief Police Officers (Home Office Digest 2004):

CANNABIS IS STILL ILLEGAL

The Police can arrest you:
If you are **Publicly** smoking Cannabis
If you **Repeatedly** offend
If Cannabis has been **Linked** to other problems in the area
If you possess Cannabis and are close to **Youth** premises e.g. schools
You will be arrested if you are aged 17 or under

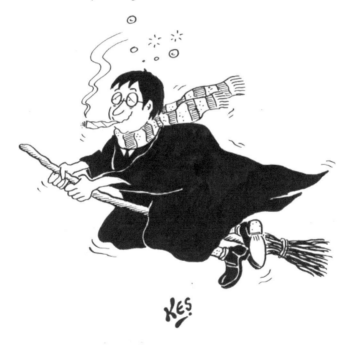

Harry Pot-head.

Credit: Cartoon Stock.com.

In fact, a survey of 15- and 16-year-old school students conducted in 2003, before reclassification occurred, examined teenagers' knowledge and opinions concerning the legal status of cannabis. The Joseph Rowntree Foundation commissioned the examination of this topic as part of the UK component of European School Survey Project on Alcohol and other Drugs (ESPAD). They also commissioned a rexamination of this subject as part of the 2007 ESPAD survey. Results from the 2003 study indicated widespread confusion about the legal status of cannabis:

- ◆ Of the 1,927 teenagers who answered the question, 959 (49.8%) thought that the reclassification of cannabis would make cannabis legal. A further 563 (27.7%) reported that they did not know. Only 405 (21.0%) correctly reported that it would remain illegal.
- ◆ The large majority 1331/1916 (69.5%) indicated that reclassification would make no difference to whether or not they used cannabis.
- ◆ Nearly half the respondents 881/1880 (46.9%) held the opinion that cannabis should be legalized in some form, 787 (41.8%) thought it should remain illegal and 212 (11.3%) either did not know or held some other view.
- ◆ A total of 461 (25.0%) felt that growing cannabis for personal use should be a more serious offence than possession of cannabis, 770 (40.8%) thought it should be equally serious and 654 (34.7%) suggested it should be a less serious offence.
- ◆ For the first three cannabis questions (beliefs regarding what the reclassification of cannabis would mean, effects of reclassification on personal cannabis use and views on whether or not cannabis should be legalised or not) family financial status, family structure, binge drinking and cigarette smoking were all totally non-significant once the effects of gender and cannabis use were controlled.

(Miller and Plant 2004, p.4)

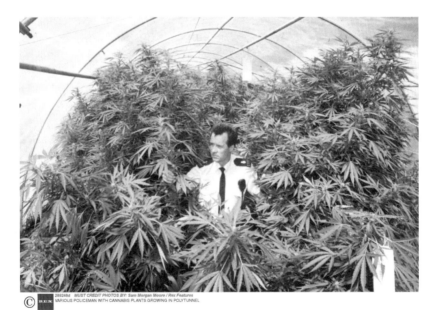

British Police officer with cannabis plants
Credit: Sam Morgan Moore/Rex Features.

The findings of the 2003 ESPAD survey were compared with those obtained in 2007. The questions used in 2007 were:

S1 Is the possession of cannabis legal? (Yes…No…Don't know)

S2 Do you think that cannabis possession should be:

    Fully legal but sold in a carefully controlled way.

    Illegal but not punished.

    Illegal and treated like a minor parking offence.

    Illegal and treated like a serious offence.

    Other (please specify).

    Don't know.

S3 Compared to possession of cannabis, should growing cannabis for personal use be:

    A more serious offence.

    An equally serious offence.

    A less serious offence.

In 2003 the Government had just announced changes to the law so that cannabis would be reclassified, downgrading it from Class B to Class C. Accordingly the first question of the 2003 ESPAD questionnaire read: 'Will these changes mean that the possession of cannabis will be… Legal…Illegal… Don't know?'. The other two questions were almost identical, thus making it possible to compare the findings for the two survey years. The response alternatives for question S2 were recoded into 'legal', 'minor offence', 'serious offence,' and 'don't know/other'. Table 8.2 shows the breakdowns of the three questions for boys and girls in the two study years.

Teenage attitudes towards cannabis were less favourable in 2007 than they had been in 2003. For instance, in 2003 just over half the boys questioned felt that cannabis should be legal (see Table 8.2), whereas in 2007 this proportion had dropped to just over one-quarter. This coincided with a fall in self-reported cannabis use over the 2 years. In 2003 cannabis had been tried at least once by 41% of boys while in 2007 the figure was 30%. For girls the decline was from 35% in 2003 to 28% in 2007.

Two continuous variables were also investigated. The first, termed 'minor delinquency', was the sum of the following five items scored 0 for no and 1 for yes:

During the last 12 months how often have you:

    used any kind of weapon to get something from a person?

    taken something not belonging to you worth over £7?

    taken something from a shop without paying for it?

Table 8.2 Beliefs about cannabis and the law for boys and girls shown by the ESPAD surveys in 2003 and 2007

Question	Gender	Response	2003	2007	χ^2
2003: will cannabis be legal? 2007: is cannabis legal?*	Boys	Yes	524 (49.6%)	336 (38.9%)	
		No	235 (36.7%)	405 (46.9%)	141.0***
		Don't know	298 (28.2%)	123 (14.2%)	
	Girls	Yes	527 (52.2%)	390 (35.5%)	
		No	160 (15.8%)	498 (45.4%)	214.7***
		Don't know	323 (32.0%)	210 (19.1%)	
Do you think cannabis possession should be:	Boys	Legal	533 (51.9%)	217 (25.6%)	
		Minor offence	207 (20.2%)	207 (24.4%)	
		Serious offence	184 (17.9%)	260 (30.7%)	144.4***
		Don't know	102 (9.9%)	163 (19.2%)	
	Girls	Legal	428 (43.2%)	197 (18.1%)	
		Minor offence	213 (21.5%)	282 (25.9%)	
		Serious offence	193 (19.5%)	337 (31.0%)	161.3***
		Don't know	156 (15.8%)	272 (25.0%)	
Compared to possession should growing cannabis for own use be:	Boys	More serious	255 (24.5%)	304 (35.9%)	
		Equally serious	375 (36.1%)	312 (36.9%)	41.2***
		Less serious	410 (39.4%)	230 (27.2%)	
	Girls	More serious	245 (25.1%)	362 (33.9%)	
		Equally serious	424 (43.4%)	501 (46.9%)	45.7***
		Less serious	308 (31.5%)	205 (19.2%)	

*See text.

*** $P<0.001$. A significant chi-square statistic indicates deviation from an equal response in the 2 years.

set fire to somebody else's property on purpose?

damaged school property on purpose?

The second, termed 'fighting', was the sum of the following three items scored 0 for no and 1 for yes:

During the last 12 months how often have you:

got mixed into a fight at school or at work?

taken part in a fight where a group of your friends were against another group?

hurt somebody badly enough to need bandages or a doctor?

Table 8.3 sets out the findings related to these two variables.

Thus it appears that there was a considerable drop between 2003 and 2007 in the proportions of teenagers who believed that cannabis should be fully legal. Even so, in 2007 the proportions believing that cannabis should be fully legal were still 25.6% among boys and 18.1% among girls. In both years teenagers in favour of legalization were to be found predominantly among those who had used cannabis and/or engaged in various types of antisocial behaviour and whose circle of friends included many who had also used cannabis. Parental attitudes were also important. Legalization was more favoured by teenagers from families in which the parents did not forbid their children to use cannabis.

The strongest association between the view on legalization and another variable was with the subject's own cannabis use. However, the difference in this regard between those who had and had not used cannabis was less in 2007 than it had been in 2003. This is shown by the interaction effect when the variables year, cannabis use, and their interaction are entered into a logistic regression equation predicting beliefs about legalization. Some of the other variables showed similar but less marked effects (parental education, father's views on cannabis, lifetime intoxication, and own tobacco smoking).

Table 8.3 Minor delinquency and fighting broken down according to beliefs concerning the legality of cannabis in 2003 and 2007

Category and year	Opinion	Mean (N)	Standard deviation	t
Minor delinquency year 2003	Cannabis should be legal	0.84 (941)	1.25	10.50***
	Cannabis should not be legal	0.34 (1048)	0.77	
Minor delinquency year 2007	Cannabis should be legal	0.97 (408)	1.27	7.6***
	Cannabis should not be legal	0.46 (1479)	0.89	
Fighting year 2003	Cannabis should be legal	0.78 (953)	1.01	8.3***
	Cannabis should not be legal	0.44 (1051)	0.80	
Fighting year 2007	Cannabis should be legal	0.78 (408)	1.03	5.4***
	Cannabis should not be legal	0.49 (1485)	0.85	

*** $P < 0.001$.

The reasons for the overall difference between the 2 years are unclear but there are some possibilities. Firstly research into the adverse effects of cannabis proceeded apace, and the dangers for a minority of users such as extreme feelings of paranoia and the triggering of schizophrenic episodes may have become more widely known (McBride and Thomas 1995, Wylie et al. 1995, Potter et al. 2008). Murray, one of the main people to have warned of the dangers of cannabis, has expressed the following view:

> It is estimated that at least 10 per cent of all people with schizophrenia in the UK would not have developed the illness if they had not smoked cannabis, so there are about 25,000 individuals whose lives have been ruined by cannabis.
> Why are we seeing so many cases of cannabis-induced schizophrenia? A UN report in 2006 suggested three reasons.
> First, the consumption of cannabis climbed steadily across Europe over the past four decades to reach a peak about 2002.
> Second, high-potency cannabis preparations are more widely available. Traditional 1960s herbal cannabis contained about 2-3 per cent of the active ingredient tetrahydrocannabinol (THC); but today's skunk varieties may contain 15 or 20 per cent THC and new resin preparations have up to 30 per cent. Skunk is to old-fashioned hash as is whisky to lager. You can become alcoholic by just drinking lager; but you have to drink a lot more lager than whisky. Similarly, you can go psychotic if you smoke enough traditional marijuana, but you have to consume a lot more for a lot longer than with skunk.
> Third, the age of starting cannabis use has been steadily lowering. It is now commonly taken at 15 and some of the patients I see started at 12 or 13 years.
> Of course, most cannabis smokers never come to any harm, just as the vast majority of drinkers don't get liver disease. It is simply that the more you take the greater the risk.
>
> (Murray 2007)

The fact that an increasing proportion of UK cannabis has been available in the form of stronger skunk has been widely publicized by the media. This could at least explain the interaction effect noted above, with more of the teenagers who tried it reporting that they did not favour legalizing cannabis.

During January 2005 the Home Office released the following positive statement related to the impact of the changed legal status of cannabis:

> Arrests for cannabis possession have fallen by one third in the first year since re-classification. This has led to an estimated saving in police time of 199,000 police hours, the Home Office announced today. Cannabis use by young people has remained stable following reclassification, and is significantly down since April 1998—28.2 per cent of 16-24 year olds used cannabis then compared to 24.8 per cent now.

> Caroline Flint said:

> "The Government's drugs strategy focuses on tackling the class A drugs which cause the most harm to communities, individuals and their families. A year ago we reclassified

cannabis on the recommendation of the ACMD, so that the police could concentrate on the far more destructive class A drugs.

"One year on the picture is encouraging with significant savings in police time which can now be used to drive more serious drugs off our streets and make our communities safer. 155 crack houses were closed by the police between January and September last year and in January we launched a national enforcement campaign, Operation Crackdown, to clamp down further on class A drugs.

"I am also pleased that figures show that some predictions that cannabis use by young people would increase were wholly unfounded. Following a major Government information campaign to get across that cannabis is harmful and remains illegal, the figures show that young people's cannabis use has remained stable since reclassification and is still significantly down from 1998 levels. We are not complacent about drugs. Illegal drug use is still too high and fuels crime and misery for individuals and neighbourhoods. That is why we are continuing to take tough action to tackle drug users, dealers and the organised criminals who supply the drugs which end up on our streets."

(Home Office Online 2005b)

Reclassify, again?

Following a request from the Home Secretary, in March 2005, the Advisory Council reconsidered its view on the still controversial classification of cannabis. A new report (Advisory Council on the Misuse of Drugs 2005) set out the following conclusions:

The Advisory Council remains of the view that cannabis is harmful and its consumption can lead to a wide range of physical and psychological hazards. Nevertheless, it does not recommend that the classification of cannabis products should be changed on the basis of the results of recent research into the effects on the development of mental illness. Although cannabis is unquestionably harmful, its harmfulness does not equate to that of other Class B substances either at the level of the individual or of society.

(Advisory Council on the Misuse of Drugs 2005)

During 2007 a fresh debate about the legal status of cannabis erupted. In July of that year the Prime Minister, Gordon Brown, ordered a review of this topic, apparently due to reports of:

warnings of links between much more potent strains coming on to the market and mental illness.

(Travis 2007)

Police chiefs have come out in support of reclassifying cannabis as a Class B drug just three years after they supported the controversial Government decision to downgrade it legally to a less serious Class C substance. Chief constables were in favour of the downgrading in 2004 because they believed it would free time spent on prosecuting cannabis users to tackle hard drugs. Their view was heavily influential in the decision by the then-Home Secretary, David Blunkett. However, they have reversed their stance because they now believe the downwards re-classification created confusion about

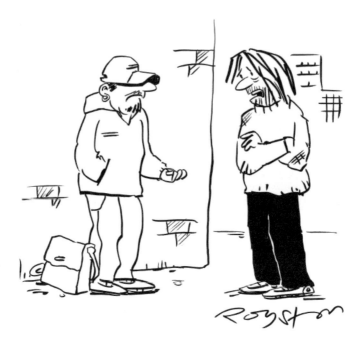

"I dunno, man, you can't be too careful these days
– do you have anything that's Class C?"

Credit: Cartoon Stock.com.

the legality of the drug in the public mind and sent the wrong signals to teenagers, who suffer most from its harmful effects.

They are also concerned that organised crime gangs have targeted the UK, establishing thousands of back-street "cannabis factories" to grow the high-strength 'skunk' version of the drug.

(Steele 2007)

The debate continued to reverberate during 2008:

Senior police are calling for cannabis to become a class B drug again after it was reported that a government advisory body will say it should remain class C.

The Superintendents' Association said downgrading the drug in 2004 had sent out the wrong message by implying cannabis was harmless and legal.

The Association of Chief Police Officers (Acpo) has also said this.

If it is reclassified, people caught carrying the drug would face up to five years in prison, rather than two…

The BBC understands the Advisory Council on the Misuse of Drugs - asked by the government to review the legal status of cannabis - will suggest it should retain its current classification.

> But it appears the recommendation will go against the view of Gordon Brown, who seems to favour returning the drug to class B.
>
> Some mental health charities have also come out in support of reclassification, voicing concerns over the strength of some forms of cannabis, in particular skunk.
>
> (BBC News Online, 3 April, 2008a)

In April 2008 a number of media reports suggested that the Government was likely to reject the ACMD's anticipated recommendation that cannabis should not be reclassified (again):

> Gordon Brown is to take personal responsibility for toughening the law on cannabis.
>
> The Prime Minister will over-rule the Government's panel of experts to announce next week that he wants it to return to Class B status. The U-turn will involve a damning admission that labour's soft policy of recent years was a mistake and will bring down the curtain on a disastrous experiment begun by Tony Blair in 2004.
>
> The shift to Class C- which meant most users faced a simple ticking off if caught-has coincided with an explosion of drug-related crime and several brutal cannabis-related murders.
>
> (Slack and Brogan 2008, p.1)

The ACMD produced its report on cannabis in October 2008. This report made 21 recommendations. The report emphasized that cannabis use was a serious public health issue. Even so, most of the Council's members agreed that cannabis should not be reclassified back to Class B on the grounds that:

> It is judged that the harmfulness of cannabis more closely equates with other Class C substances than with those currently classified as Class B.
>
> (Advisory Council on the Misuse of Drugs 2008, p.1)

The report was immediately attacked by both Conservative and Labour politicians (some of whom had even been attacking it in advance of publication). Its recommendation concerning the reclassification of cannabis was rejected by Prime Minister Gordon Brown. The Government ignored the advice of the ACMD. Cannabis again became a Category B drug in the UK in January 2009. A study of public attitudes conducted in 2007 had indicated that 58% of those surveyed believed that taking cannabis should remain illegal (National Centre for Social Research 2010).

Much of the anxiety and opposition to redefining the position and criminal justice attitude towards cannabis comes from outside the UK. North America has a longstanding hostility to cannabis which is complex in its origins and overlaps with its historic relationships with its southern neighbour Mexico. Control of cannabis importation has always been high on the agenda for the USA and in the early part of the twentieth century cannabis and cannabis users were demonized and portrayed as a major threat to the American way of life.

Within the United Nations the USA and other countries, notably Sweden, have espoused an authoritarian approach to cannabis control. This was evident during the recent changes in the UK and may well have had some influence on the 2009 decision to return cannabis to Class B with the associated increase in sentencing tariffs.

It is apparent that the Misuse of Drugs Act, although a piece of domestic UK legislation, defers to international treaties and conventions and that proposed changes have to recognize this influence. It is also clear that changes or proposed improvements based on science or evidence of relative harms are secondary in the minds of legislators and politicians to political concerns.

Ecstasy

Ecstasy (MDMA) is another drug the classification of which has been controversial. The debate on this subject has been highly emotive, overshadowed by media deathbed images of Leah Betts, an 18-year-old woman who allegedly died because she had used ecstasy. As noted in Chapter 5, the Runciman Report by the Police Foundation recommended that both ecstasy and LSD should be moved from Class A to Class B (Police Foundation 2000). Another report by the Science and Technology Committee of the House of Commons made a similar recommendation. This committee had received evidence suggesting that ecstasy was a low-risk drug that did not warrant its Class A status (Science and Technology Committee 2006). Nutt et al. (2007) had reported that ecstasy was one of the least dangerous or harmful of drugs, and was, for example, less dangerous than alcohol or tobacco. During May 2008 David Nutt became Chairman of the ACMD. His appointment was viewed by some as reopening the case for the reclassification of ecstasy, and it was announced in September 2008 that the ACMD would review the drug's status. The Committee reported on this subject in February 2009. Their report was preceded by leaks indicating that the ACMD favoured reclassifying ecstasy (then a Category A drug) to Category B. The publication of the committee's report was preceded by the bizarre spectacle of David Nutt being harangued by the indignant then Home Secretary, Jacqui Smith, who strongly opposed reclassification. She criticized David Nutt's widely quoted comparison (in a scientific journal) of the dangers of taking ecstasy with those of riding a horse (or 'equasy') (Nutt 2009a). He was, she claimed, trivializing the dangers of the drug. It was remarkable to see a senior member of a government that had committed itself to being guided by evidence attacking not only its chief drug adviser, an internationally acknowledged drug expert, but also the findings of its own scientific advisory committee. The latter concluded from a detailed and balanced review of evidence that ecstasy was not as dangerous as other substances in Category A and should be downgraded to Category B (Advisory Council on the Misuse of Drugs 2009a). Smith justified her opposition to ecstasy reclassification on the grounds that it would 'send the wrong signal'. She suggested that David Nutt should apologize to the 'families and victims of ecstasy' (Leith 2009). The reclassification debate had now clearly become a collision between rationality and irrationality. The clash between science and politics was just about to erupt into outright warfare.

Who determines policy?

ACMD chairman David Nutt produced a paper entitled 'Estimating Drug Harms: a Risky Business?' (Nutt 2009b) This document criticized the artificial separation of alcohol and tobacco from illicit drugs. Nutt pointed out that the classification of drugs had become politicized. He also noted that 'there is a relatively small risk for smoking cannabis and psychotic illness compared with quite a substantial risk of smoking tobacco and lung cancer'. He also noted:

> A fully scientifically-based Misuse of Drugs Act where drug classification accurately reflects harms would be a powerful educational tool. Using the Act in a political way to give messages other than those relating to relative harms undermines the Act and does great damage to the educational message.

> (Nutt 2009b, p.12)

Nutt's analysis, which included a defence of the ACMD's view that cannabis should not be restored as a Category B drug, clearly infuriated some people. The Home Secretary Alan Johnson, in a move that shocked and horrified most of the scientific community, sent David Nutt an e-mail dismissing him from his unpaid position as Chairman of the ACMD. Johnson informed Nutt that he had lost confidence in Nutt's ability to give impartial advice. Some people have interpreted this as implying that Alan Johnson did not want David Nutt or anybody else to provide honest information to the public about the respective harms associated with alcohol, tobacco, and illicit drugs. David Nutt has since responded, stating that Gordon Brown, the Prime Minister, was guilty of making inaccurate and exaggerated statements about the dangers of cannabis, including the suggestion that it was 'lethal'.

The dismissal of David Nutt received considerable publicity, both within the UK and overseas. The core of this issue was not simply debate about the dangers of cannabis. This was a big international story because the relationship between scientific advice and public policy are important issues with world-wide relevance. It was reported that Science Minister Lord Drayson was 'appalled' by Nutt's dismissal (Wooding 2009). In addition five other members of the ACMD resigned in protest. The implications of this incident appear to have had an impact on the general position of government scientific advisors. It has been reported that the latter was under review:

> The government is to rework the terms of engagement for using scientific advice, science minister Paul Drayson has confirmed. Drayson says that the government will endorse the recommendations set out by a group of scientists in Principles for the Treatment of Independent Scientific Advice and that a set of rules governing science advisory bodies will be prepared by Christmas.
>
> (Hood 2009a, p.1)

An impressive group of senior scientists and scientific advisers issued a detailed response to the dismissal of David Nutt. Their response set out principles which, they recommended, should govern the relationship between government and its scientific advisors. These principles related to protecting academic freedom, the independence of advisors and the proper consideration of advice:

> Principles for the Treatment of Independent Scientific Advice
> 1. Academic Freedom
>   ♦ Becoming a member of an independent advisory committee does not reduce the freedom of an adviser to communicate publicly, whether via scholarly publishing and conferences, through the general media or to parliament, subject to the restrictions in existing Codes of Practice, notably:
>   • respecting confidentiality
>   • not claiming to speak for the Government, and
>   • making clear whether they are communicating on behalf of their committees
> 2. Independence of Operation
>   ♦ Independent scientific advisory bodies are protected from political and other interference in their work
>   ♦ In the context of independent scientific advice, disagreement with Government policy and the public articulation and discussion of relevant evidence and issues by members of advisory committees cannot be grounds for criticism or dismissal
>   ♦ Advisory committees need the service of an independent press office
> 3. Proper Consideration of Advice
>   ♦ Reports will normally be published and will not be criticised or rejected prior to publication
>   ♦ If the Government is minded to reject a recommendation, the relevant scientific advisory committee will normally be invited to comment privately before a final decision is made
>   ♦ It is recognised that some policy decisions are contingent on factors other than the scientific evidence, but when expert scientific advice is rejected the reasons should be described explicitly and publicly
>   ♦ The advice of expert committees does not cease to be valid merely because it is rejected or not reflected in policy-making
>
> (Sense about Science 2009)

Much of the discussion surrounding the dismissal of David Nutt was couched in reasonable terms, regardless of viewpoint. Sadly some was not. The Home Office announced on 13 January 2010 that a new ACMD chairman had been appointed to succeed David Nutt. This individual, an existing ACMD member, was retired Oxford University Professor Les Iverson, a specialist in pharmacology. Iverson is on record as expressing the view that cannabis had been wrongly classed as a dangerous drug for nearly 50 years. It was, he had stated one of the safer recreational substances, whose dangers had sometime been exaggerated.

David Nutt's response to his dismissal as ACMD chair was to form a new body, the Independent Council on Drug Harms, launched in January 2010. This new entity included several people who were past or current members of the ACMD. Nutt commented that his group was 'very powerful' and stated that it would 'tell the truth' about drugs. He also declared that the new group would produce independent scientific advice about drug effects. It would, he believed, take over this role from the ACMD. The ACMD, Nutt maintained, was no longer a credible scientific body, comprising drug-treatment specialists, police, and magistrates who would focus on policy. Nutt's new group had secured support for an initial 3 years from a hedge-fund manager, Toby Jackson, as well as the Centre for Crime and Justice Studies think tank. This radical new development has created an obvious rivalry between the badly wounded and depleted ACMD and an influential group of scientists.

Opinions are likely to continue to be offered on the subject of the best way of classifying drugs. One issue is how the different aspects of drug effects are to be weighted (Brown 2010, Nutt, 2010). In a complex area where the use of drugs takes on a greater significance than that relating to the medical and social consequences, opinion will always be varied and at times extreme and polarized. New drugs and new drug side effects and complications will test any system of classification. A report by Morgan et al. (2010) has indicated that drug users classify the relative dangers of drugs in much the same way as 'experts', but that people in general do not. These authors conclude that the public would seem to be little influenced by the classification of the Misuse of Drugs Act.

Professor Nutt's proposed system of classification of the drugs currently controlled under the Misuse of Drugs Act and the United Nation's conventions on drug control has drawn attention to the complexity and controversial nature of drug legislation. The regulations, as they stand, are presented as a system of controls based on the dangers of these drugs and their potential for harm. Whereas this is undoubtedly true, heroin is a dangerous drug, as is cocaine and all the substances included in the classification. There is, however, a greater issue at stake in these rules for politicians, legislators, and international controls. These issues are a mixture of social control, political expediency, and historical baggage. Having set up a mechanism for control and in the face of a rising population of drug users and an increasingly embedded illegal organization, alterations are fraught with political and organizational difficulties. Worse than that even minor alterations in domestic legislation can give rise to international tensions and potential disputes which rival other areas of major intergovernmental stress. The recent attempt in the UK to make a minor repositioning of cannabis in the Misuse of Drugs Act is an example of this. A small alteration effectively caused an international debate and a national tension quite disproportionate to the reality of the legal issue. Major restructuring is therefore problematic and for some countries like the USA and Sweden an issue which raises considerable ire.

From the purely superficial view of the restructuring process under the practical banner of degrees of harm there are also difficulties. Undoubtedly more people die from the effects of alcohol and tobacco than from the toxicity of heroin or cocaine and the numbers dying from the effects of ecstasy are small. There are however, as the Nutt classification shows, reasons why some drugs are more represented in the mortality figures than others. Heroin is often injected, increasing the harm potential very greatly, but alcohol is available on every street corner and its consumption is positively encouraged in many Western societies. Tobacco is a highly addictive drug whereas the addictive properties of some controlled drugs have been exaggerated in the past. Use, and therefore damage, depends on more than just the properties of the drugs: fashion, trends, availability, and convention all have a powerful influence on harm done.

If restructuring of the Misuse of Drugs Act is to be attempted then wider considerations are important: other less tasteful influences exist, political expediency seems a benign force (although it is not) compared to commercial pressures, and corruption in high places, and all these determine progress, or lack thereof. The interests of the drug black market have been equated to the size of the 'white' economy and it would be naive to believe that all these interests are well motivated; they are malignant and hostile. It certainly will take a powerful, confident, and motivated statesperson to adopt drug reform as a political platform.

Chapter 9

Therapeutic options

For anyone who has ever had a problem controlling their drug intake or who has been involved with providing therapy for drug users it is clear that treatment is complicated. There is no simple measure or message defining treatment which can be easily described in a short statement or even a short chapter. If there was, dependence or addiction as we know it might not exist. Problem drug use exists as much because relapse is often viewed as inevitable as because drugs are addictive. Treatment, therefore, is inevitably inadequate and unsatisfactory, something which successive generations of drug users, therapists, and politicians have to learn and have to find disappointing.

However, treatment and interventions do exist and are widely promoted and, in some circumstances and for some individuals, can be extremely effective. The difficulty arises from the many addictive substances available, the complexity of the individual's situation and personal ability to respond and the jungle of political and regulatory circumstances in which the individual exists. Treatment also requires an end point, a result, or—for some—a cure. Defining this end point becomes part of the discussion about the nature, content, and expectations of the process of therapeutic involvement.

Options for treatment depend, therefore, on the characteristics of the individual, the drug or drugs involved, and the environment in which he or she finds themselves. Zinberg's paradigm of 'drug, set and setting' remains as relevant as when first coined in the 1980s (Zinberg 1984). The three important features governing the impact of being an addict are the characteristics of the drug (the drug), the environment in which it is being used (the setting), and the personal features of the individual involved (the individual). All three elements are important when considering treatment interventions.

Describing treatment types and modalities often follows a pattern of listing by success rates or by availability. In some sources treatments are given by drug type. Some treatments are drug-specific: treatments for alcohol, opiates, or stimulants for example. Others see interventions as generic, applying to all addictions and recognizing the frequent presence of dependence on more than one or several substances. Treatments might be reported by success or failure and frequency of positive outcomes and it is often noted that our failure to have adequate results on which such a table or chart could be constructed represents a major fault in the system of audit and research. The preferred term, management, rather than treatment, clearly reflects the requirement for a structured approach to treatment to deal with a long-standing problem with multiple causes and distinct needs and individual requirements. Treatments overlap and may be either repeated or continuous in time. They may be specific, targeted, and contained in a package of therapy or may be supportive and general, addressing issues which sometimes seem to be peripheral to the central drug problem. They may be residential, and consequently expensive, or they may be delivered along with other services at home or in the community. They may be conducted by experts with specific knowledge of the field, by generic workers, or even by family or friends. Often apparently unrelated issues and problems may have to be addressed before drug treatment can be considered.

This chapter will consider various treatments and will review their popularity and any evidence for their efficacy. In line with contemporary thinking attempts to rate successes using simple measures such as abstinence or cure from addictive symptoms will be avoided most of the time as these measures have been shown to be inadequate and an oversimplification of a complex problem. It is also true to say that rigorous research into the cause and effect of treatment has been difficult when the outcome measure is unclear and several 'treatments' may be happening to the individual concerned over a long period of time. That is not to say that abstinence is not achievable and that cure is unheard of so much as to recognize the difficulty in saying when abstinence is an enduring state and when cure is irreversible. Research into this area has been particularly difficult for these reasons. Management will be described, therefore, using the research literature for support taking into account the benefits of interventions without the expectation that individual therapies are mutually exclusive in time or content. Most drug-dependent individuals sample many treatment modalities, often over a period of many years, and derive partial results and benefits from many of them. Improvement or recovery, partial or complete, can sometimes be attributed in retrospect to a specific intervention but more likely is seen as a cumulative response to serial or continuous supports. The expectation in this chapter will not therefore be to describe dramatically effective therapies which are superior to all others but to present the range of interventions, with all their inadequacies and imperfections, and to try to explore the complex interactions between therapy, personal development, and maturing and that miasma of other influences which negatively affect the lives of some people and which reinforces negative behaviours. Negative forces come in many forms in many lives and the effects of poverty, deprivation, adverse childhood experiences, and perhaps some genetically inherited factors are included, although there are many other contenders. Similarly positive and life-enhancing experiences come in many shapes and sizes and individually or by process of accumulation change behaviour in an improving direction. Recovered individuals will often say that a single life event turned their addiction problem around. A relationship, a birth, or a death, a period in rehabilitation, or a connection with an effective drug worker or agency are all at times given credit for forms of recovery. Equally common is the experience that a series or collection of life changes coming together give rise to a change and individuals will often say that, 'the time had come in their life to change' or that 'things had become so bad that a change had to happen'. Others will, in a more vague way, say that they had grown out of or away from their drug-using days, a sort of maturing process.

Without trying to complicate treatment, therefore, it is important to view interventions in the context of the complexities of an individual life and to understand that, like many life experiences, responses to treatments unfold over time rather than happen in an instant.

Natural history of dependency

In order to understand the efficacy and appropriateness of therapeutic interventions it is important to have some understanding of the probabilities of success and the reasons why therapy might result in a favourable outcome and what might inhibit treatment and hence interfere with recovery. That there might be a clear process in the life course of a 'disease' such as dependency has attracted researchers for many years and attempts in the literature to describe an unfolding progression in dependent individuals have been many. In studies of both alcohol and opiate addictions and dependency, as well as addictions to other substances and behaviours such as gambling, there have been many descriptions of a remitting and relapsing disorder, of successes in promoting abstinence and of causes of relapse. There are classic accounts of cohorts divided into several groups of individuals who exhibit similar patterns of drug taking and which differ from each other. Both alcohol and opiate studies show individual types who can sample addictive substances and then abstain, apparently for ever, while other groups fall into categories of frequent relapsers or binge users. Another, apparently larger, group seems to pursue an unrelenting path of dependent substance misuse and a third sector of any study demonstrates the up and down pattern of remission and relapse over many years (Kimber et al. 2010). Although attempts to define these groups by personality or experiential characteristics have been less successful there are many associations which contribute to success, abstinence, relapse, or persistent use. It is easy to imagine, for example, how associated mental health problems, concurrent HIV or hepatitis C infection, or social disintegration might precipitate crises and how positive life events might enhance or precipitate recovery.

Many countries are exploring the impact of illicit drug-use treatment and the implications for treatment. Evidence is available and is accumulating from countries in Western Europe and Australia to show the stabilizing effects of methadone treatment and the relative benefits to controlling criminal behaviour and reducing the incidence of HIV and other blood-borne virus transmission. In the UK, Germany, France, and the Netherlands HIV prevalence has stabilized, decreased, or failed to increase as might be expected in the absence of these interventions (Hamers et al. 1997, Wodak et al. 1996, Nadelmann et al. 1997). The Netherlands has had the most consistent and long-standing policy on methadone provision and needle and syringe provision and Germany from a relatively late start in the 1990s has shown rapid growth and impact of these services. Scotland was perhaps the first country to establish a formal national policy on the supply of injecting equipment (Scottish Home and Health Department 1986) but has shown recent signs of widening policy objectives raising concerns of dilution of basic harm-minimization programmes (Scottish Government 2008). In Canada worrying trends are reported and linked to relatively slow public health support for methadone programmes (Fischer et al. 1997). Estimates of HIV prevalence among injecting drug users were available for 84 out of 192 United Nations member states and reported to be more than 25% in Argentina, Brazil, Estonia, Indonesia, Kenya, Myanmar (Burma), Nepal, Puerto Rico, Spain, Tanzania, Thailand, and Uruguay (Mathers et al. 2008).

Definitions are important in this chapter on treatment. Without being sure of the nature of the disorder treatment is hard to construct and in the absence of a clear understanding and terminology for recovery and improvement it is difficult to measure or recognize it when it happens.

Addiction is a term of general use but is defined in scientific terms in international medical terminology in various publications (*International Classification of Diseases ICD 10* (World Health Organization 1994) and *Diagnostic and Statistical Manual of Mental Disorders* (DSM) IV, published in APA 2000). Most definitions of addiction contain three important components: the presence of physical or psychological dependence or craving, the associated presence of tolerance to the drug in question, and the presence of withdrawal symptoms when use is discontinued.

Recovery is not a clinical term or a word that has a strict definition in the context of addictions but various attempts have been made to describe what it is. Two examples come from the UK Drug Policy Commission and the US Betty Ford Institute and both have a similar approach:

> The process of recovery is characterised by voluntary sustained control over substance use which maximises health and well-being and participation in the rights, roles and responsibilities of society.
>
> (UK Drug Policy Commission 2008)

> ...voluntary maintained lifestyle comprised of sobriety, personal health and citizenship...
>
> (Letter to editor Betty Ford Institute Panel 2009)

Detoxification is a familiar term to most people although it often means different things depending upon the context in which it is used. In the context of drug dependence detoxification is the process of managing the removal of the drug from the system, a process which will happen with little interference by anyone as the substance in question is metabolized over time in the liver. Support given during this process by medical or other support agencies can be more, or less, intensive. Programmes of detoxification range from intensive medical interventions with sedation and alternative medications, to emotional social and psychological support only with no pharmaceutical intervention. Success often depends on personal factors as much as the intensity of the intervention.

Rehabilitation is generally seen as a longer process of adjustment to a drug-free or a controlled drug intake and can take many forms. Programmes which support rehabilitation are often residential and contain social psychological and practical help. Others are community-based or domestic. Time factors are variable and can be short or many months. Length of time taken to rehabilitate depends on personal circumstances as well as drug-related factors and programmes are often arbitrarily time-limited due to cost factors.

Harm minimization, otherwise known as risk reduction, is as much a philosophical approach as it is a programme or distinctive process. At the individual level harm minimization is often applied to an educational and support process to reduce the risks involved with drug taking. This might be the engagement with a drug user to avoid injecting, reducing injecting, or simply eliminating sharing of equipment. A hierarchy of objectives and associated interventions are included in Table 9.1, which demonstrates various objectives which may be identified and attempted and the interventions that might support them.

Table 9.1 Harm minimization: hierarchy of targets for improvement

Goal	Intervention
Stop unsafe injecting	Needle exchange
Stop injecting	Change subculture
Stop illicit drug use	Substitute prescribing
Normalize lifestyle	Maintenance prescribing
Stop drug use	Withdrawal programmes

The concept of harm minimization or risk reduction is not new but became acceptable to many healthcare workers and policy makers at the time of the introduction of HIV infection. Even though hepatitis B had for many years been recognized as a hazard for those engaged in drug use it was only the imperative of preventing HIV spread that focused attention on needle and syringe sharing and gave rise to serious consideration for prevention. The realization that abstinence was, at least in the short term, unachievable for many drug users allowed the development of a multifaceted line of intervention. This included provision of injecting equipment, prescription opiate drugs, and health education and counselling. The notion that reducing harm in itself must be good is intuitively correct although in its simplest form it is seen by some as minimalist, unaspirational, or—worse still—a negative and neglectful lack of commitment to a better and more serious treatment. It is true that to aspire to raising a chaotic lifestyle from the bottom rung to the next one up may be uninspiring but using the example again of blood-borne virus transmission, the quintessentially harm-minimalization approach of providing injecting equipment may, and has, saved many lives and perhaps prevented epidemic transmission. Clearly, faced with a chaotic and vulnerable individual, minimizing the harm makes perfect sense. Similarly methadone treatment and even long-term methadone or other opiate treatment can be seen as a minimizing the harm intervention and one with a substantial evidence base which shows its efficacy. For many observers this is not enough. Proper treatment must try harder and be leading the individual progressively in a direction towards a serious change in lifestyle; strategies are being investigated to develop improvement in circumstances, even towards abstinence from drugs and it seems sensible to embrace all ideas in this direction. Harm-reduction schemes may also offer the following:

- a needle exchange operates by providing sterile injecting equipment to injecting drug users and disposing of used injecting equipment, with the aim of reducing infection;
- immunization against hepatitis B;

- information on the prevention of infection from blood-borne diseases, such as HIV and hepatitis B and C;
- advice and information on HIV, hepatitis, and drug problems;
- advice and information on overdose prevention/response, safer sex, and sexual health;
- provide referral to other treatment services.

A hierarchy of targets for improvements are set out in Table 9.1.

Management of opiate-dependency problems

Although there is no shortage of literature on this topic there have been some very useful additions in recent years. Much of what is needed by those treating patients or researching the background to treatment is available in a recent document from the National Institute for Health and Clinical Excellence (NICE). The document entitled *Methadone and Buprenorphine for the Treatment of Opioid Dependence* (National Institute for Health and Clinical Excellence 2007d) confirms the efficacy of these treatments and reports on the supporting literature. Similarly the updated Department of Health's *Drug Misuse and Dependence: UK Guidelines on Clinical Management* enhances the field by elaborating on many aspects of drug treatment including comments on many modalities of treatment and the alternatives available (Department of Health 2007). This latter document is the definitive source for clinicians working in the UK National Health Service and provides more than just guidelines, giving a clear and detailed account of most of the pragmatic ways to manage the wide range of issues encountered by drug dependents.

Clinical management of drug-dependent patients is inevitably complicated by the range of problems experienced in the course of drug use and associated with a drug-using lifestyle. Table 9.2 lists some of the complications encountered and divides them into issues occurring at different junctures in a drug-using career. These are for guidance only and clearly most of these problems can occur at any stage but for this discussion it is useful to note that problems are episodic and sometimes cumulative and most importantly are preventable with early interventions. When considering opiate-dependency treatment the assumption is that heroin is the drug to which the individual is addicted and that this is the problem to be treated. There is, however, a wide range of opiates which are misused, many of them pharmaceutically prepared. These include codeine and codeine-containing compound drugs, oxycodone and preparations which contain it, buprenorphine and methadone which have been diverted from treatment prescriptions, hydromorphone, dipipanone, and other rarely prescribed opiates which may be available through illegal

Table 9.2 The problems associated with drug use as they emerge over time from early experiences to long-term use

Time of life	Problem
Problems which may be experienced in early months or years of drug use	Hepatitis A, B, and C
	HIV infection
	Overdose
	Endocarditis
	Superficial venous infections
	Soft-tissue infections
	Violent incidents
Problems for drug takers when they become regular users	Social difficulties
	Unemployment
	Relationship and family problems
	Treatment sampling with variable success and frequent failures
	Prison
	Remission and relapse is common
Issues for drug users as they become older and accumulate problems and as various diseases progress	Progression of blood-borne virus diseases which may have been contracted many years before
	Depression and overdose: the latter sometimes due to injudicious withdrawal from medications
	Arterial and deep-vein problems
	Venous access problems
	Advancing liver disease causing loss of tolerance
	Alcohol problems, self neglect, and tuberculosis
	Premature old age (premature cardiovascular and respiratory disorders)

pharmaceutical channels. Treatment for all opiate problems is similar and there is some evidence to show that the same interventions are appropriate. Comparing the key parameter of retention in treatment Banta-Green and colleagues (2009) found no significant difference, and concluded that the data suggest that prescription-type opioid primary users can be treated at methadone-maintenance treatment facilities at least as effectively as heroin users.

Types of treatment

This section is modified from a DrugScope webpage (www.drugscope.org.uk/resources/databases/typesoftreatment). In the *Models of Care* document (National Treatment Agency for Substance Misuse 2002) there is described a tiered system of treatment modalities available in England and Wales. This is a means of classifying drug-treatment services in a way that is easy to understand. Each drug-treatment provider in this database is classified according to which modality it belongs, and the list clearly identifies the enormity of the responses required to provide care and treatment in the realms of drug and alcohol problems.

Tiers of drug treatment provision

Tier 1: Non-specific (general) service

> General practitioners (general medical services)

> Probation

> Housing

Tier 2: Open access service

> Advice and information

> Drop-in service

> Harm-reduction services

Tier 3: Community services

> Community drug teams

> Drug-dependency units

> Day treatment

Tier 4a: Specialist services (residential)

> Inpatient

> Residential rehabilitation

Tier 4b: Highly specialist (non-substance misuse) services

> Liver units

> Forensic services

Pharmacological interventions

The most common pharmacotherapy in the UK concerns substituting an opioid substitute (usually oral methadone) for illicit heroin. To be effective it must be given at a level that will prevent the onset of withdrawal symptoms and maintain a feeling of stability. Pharmacotherapy for dependent users of amphetamines is also available, albeit less common. There is currently no pharmacotherapy aimed at cocaine and crack cocaine dependence although trials are going ahead of candidate drugs.

In UK policy it is recommended that community prescribing takes place in a context within which the coexisting physical, emotional, social, and legal problems are addressed as far as possible. Community prescribing services offer the provision of medically supervised substitutes to misusers of illicit drugs based on recent Department of Health (2007) guidelines, which stressed the importance of a shared care approach between primary (general practitioners) and secondary care (specialist drug treatment) in the management of drug misusers.

General practitioners are encouraged to provide specialist treatment programmes which may involve them prescribing substitutes. They are also encouraged not to prescribe in isolation but to liaise with other professionals who will help with factors contributing to drug misuse. A multidisciplinary approach to treatment is therefore essential.

Methadone

Methadone is an effective maintenance therapy intervention for the treatment of heroin dependence as it retains patients in treatment and decreases heroin use better than treatments that do not utilize opioid-replacement therapy. For some reason this simple statement fails to convince politicians, the public, and serial generations of healthcare professionals who require repeated and detailed evidence. Research has, however, been consistent and cumulative over more than three decades to demonstrate the efficacy and relative popularity of this treatment. Continual refining of treatment delivery has shown that there is a patient variability in acceptance of methadone treatment and a spectrum of delivery of the treatment to suit a variable population of opiate-dependent individuals. Not all patients are tolerant of an opiate medication like methadone; they may find it over-sedating or that it causes nausea or dysphoria and others find that they require a larger dose than average to have the desired effect. Its effect is to replace the need for the shorter-acting heroin with a long-acting drug which occupies the same neurological receptors in the central nervous system. At high dose its effect is described in the original research as a 'narcotic blockade' and this description has become the popular explanation for its mode of action. With a half-life of more than 24 h a single daily dose is usually enough to remove craving and to eliminate the withdrawal symptoms present when a short-acting drug such as injectable heroin is used. Clearly the effect of a longer, slow-onset treatment loses the desirable sudden 'rush' euphoria of a short-acting drug delivered by venous injection but for those with any motivation the transition from the illegal 'high' to a legal, available, and free medication is attractive in both the short-term and certainly in the longer-term control of a dependency problem.

Methadone has its dangers. A drug with a slow onset it can, for the first-time user, seem innocuous and safe when first taken but its cumulative effect over several days makes the induction period hazardous, especially if the continued use of additional opiates, sedatives, or alcohol is not avoided. In the longer-term periods of abstinence brought about by loss of access to the drug or by custodial removal from its availability can result in loss of tolerance and subsequent overdose when recommencing the previous level of intake. At any stage the additional use of other drugs can precipitate an overdose situation or loss of capacity to metabolize the drug when, for example, liver function is impaired.

One of the single most important factors in safe and successful treatment with methadone is an adequate assessment of drug use and general health at onset of treatment. This requires some skill, experience, and attention to details but need not necessarily be complex or excessively time-consuming. Establishing the urgency and importance of treatment can be deduced by clinical observation of the damage done by injecting and the intensity of the dependency by the domestic and personal situation of the patient. The presence of withdrawal symptoms need not necessarily be a determinant of the need to commence treatment as these may have been present off and on for months or years in the lifestyle of the individual. Present and persistent illegal drug taking in a more or less risky fashion makes treatment a matter of urgency. Similarly, the presence of a crisis such as lack of available illegal opiate or an impending court case may not indicate a commitment to engaging in treatment. The purpose of methadone treatment is to replace a need to buy illegal heroin in a person with a resolution to change to a more controlled life. Further assessment includes the risks taken over the time of injecting drug use of acquiring a blood-borne virus, the general health state, and the domestic social and financial situation present. All these factors may indicate the need for additional medical or social interventions or the presence, or absence, of a family infrastructure or domestic comforts. Commencing methadone treatment is usually carried out using a local or national protocol and guideline.

Delivery of a treatment like methadone or other opiate substitute such as buprenorphine requires a robust service with the capacity to carry out assessments, the ability to prescribe, and the flexibility to monitor treatment over months and years. This is done in partnership with medical, psychiatric, pharmacy, and social services and requires the investment of an agency with long-term support and year-round availability.

Drug testing is an essential, but possibly overrated, component of the service. Confirmation of the presence in a urine, blood, or oral fluid sample is extremely useful prior to treatment and the periodic assessment of compliance with treatment and the use of non-prescribed drugs may be a useful guideline as to the success or lack of adequacy of the treatment. When used excessively as a means of coercion repeated testing can be counterproductive.

Opiate and other treatment services are not expected to consist of pharmacological interventions alone. Evidence has long been available to show that the addition of talking therapies and support programmes enhance the results of methadone and other substitute prescribing. Examples of so-called add on services are structured counselling, structured day programmes: and aftercare. Structured counselling is defined as formal counselling approached with assessment, clearly defined treatment plans and treatment goals, and regular reviews. It is distinct from advice and information, drop-in support, and informal key-working. Structured day programmes: drug-treatment providers in this category offer intensive community-based support, treatment, and rehabilitation. Programmes of defined activities for a fixed period of time will be on offer and will require a specific level of attendance, usually 4–5 days a week. Aftercare drug-treatment services provide structured support for clients on exit from another programme. The development of an appropriate package of aftercare and support should take place in the final phase of the treatment episode of service users aiming to achieve abstinence.

Opiate substitutes are obviously only useful as a therapy for those using this category of drug. There are, however, treatments common to all drugs of addiction and usually required in addition to the pharmacological approach. These come under the general heading of psychosocial interventions and can include a variety of types of intervention ranging from counselling and cognitive behavioural therapy to more intensive treatments of serious mental health problems. A wide range of social supports and support group treatments are described in the literature. As part of the general assessment procedure the therapist is on the look out for a therapy or treatment option which might be matched to the personal or individual need of the patient. An underlying past experience of sexual abuse in childhood, a coexisting anxiety state, a personal risk of assault from a violent partner, or a homeless person might all be indications that additional agency help is needed.

Detoxification and rehabilitation

Detoxification and rehabilitation can be part of the same process, one leading on to the other over a shorter or longer period. The process of detoxification implies a short episode of getting over the effects of withdrawal from a drug and the period during which the drug and its metabolites are removed from the body. This is essentially a natural biological activity during which the drug is metabolized in the liver into metabolic products, some of which may be psychoactive themselves, and the elimination of these products by excretion from the kidneys. This length of time the process takes depends on the pharmacokinetics of the drug and the pharmacodynamics of the host. Some drugs persist in the body longer than others and some people have a slower metabolic make-up, leading to a longer period of elimination. The duration of the detoxification time is difficult to alter but medical and support interventions are commonly offered to mitigate the pain and discomfort of the withdrawal experience. Depending upon the drug or drugs involved, sedatives, tranquillizers, and medications to reduce nausea or convulsions may be administered or a longer-acting substitute given with gradual reduction over a prolonged period. The additional presence of sympathetic surroundings and psychological support are important, as can be the physical removal from the environment in which the addiction is encouraged. The model of a short-stay residential facility with social, psychological, and medical support is that commonly envisaged for managing the detoxification process. This model takes no account, however, of the psychological drives to recommence illegal drug taking. The evidence shows that the majority of abstinence attempts result in relapse and the need to link detoxification with a longer, more intensive, rehabilitation treatment programme becomes apparent.

Inpatient detoxification programmes are specialized units for people with substance misuse disorders, which provide medically supervised withdrawal with 24-hour medical cover (and usually relapse prevention) and aftercare referral services. Rehabilitation programmes come in many shapes and sizes and residential sessions can last for periods of usually not less than 3 months but may extend to more than a year. These drug-treatment providers offer intensive and structured programmes in controlled residential or hospital inpatient environments. Some crisis-intervention services have open access; others require formal referral via a health or social care agency. Rehabilitation services vary in approach programme structure, intensity, and duration. The majority of residential rehabilitation services require users to be drug-free on entry, although some may have on-site detoxification facilities.

At first sight these treatments—detoxification and rehabilitation—for drug dependency must seem to be the most sensible intervention and for most observers, if not people with the addiction problem, it may be a surprise to hear that these are not the first and only treatments of choice. Abstinence-related treatments are relatively poorly available, not supported by appropriate central funding streams, and are often not chosen by drug users. For families, relatives, and the public this approach to the problems of drugs users is, intuitively, the correct one. Reluctance to fund such expensive interventions is not surprising and the high failure rate makes cost-effectiveness an issue. Careful selection and preparation of participants to maximize benefits is essential.

On the topic of detoxification and rehabilitation the conclusion of one review publication (Simoens et al. 2002) was as follows:

- a wide range of different models of community detoxification have been studied;
- relapse rates range from 19% to 83%;
- alpha adrenergic agonists are reasonably effective at relieving withdrawal symptoms and, thus, improve outcomes;
- lofexidine appears to be slightly more effective at reducing withdrawal symptoms and, importantly, has considerably less adverse effects on blood pressure than clonidine;
- buprenorphine could have an important role in detoxification but further U.K.-based studies are required;
- the role of methadone appears to be limited in detoxification as it was associated with particularly high drop-out rates;
- counselling/behavioural treatment is associated with improved outcomes.

Future studies need to focus on the longer term follow-up of clients enrolled in a detoxification programme and on the support and counselling part of detoxification interventions.

(Simoens et al. 2002, p.49)

And on the subject of residential rehabilitation:

- residential rehabilitation is effective in terms of reduction in illicit opiate use, employment status, risk behaviours, and crime rates;
- retention in and completion of treatment are more important than length of treatment in influencing outcomes;
- residential rehabilitation programmes that provide more health and treatment services and encourage client participation are more effective.

There is an urgent need for better-designed studies on the effectiveness of the various residential rehabilitation programmes in the U.K.

(Simoens et al. 2002, p.58)

Treatment of drug-use complications and associated problems

Associated with the problems of the dependency being treated there are often added complexities. These may be coexisting medical or social problems or other addictions. The list below contains examples of comorbidities and situations which may influence treatment. Often several of these coexisting states or conditions are present and contribute to the difficulties associated with recovery and rehabilitation. Increasingly, long-standing, older drug users are requiring treatment for several conditions at the same time, thus clearly increasing the challenge to the individual and the treatment service. It is likely that in the future multidimensional treatment services will be required with the capability of delivering medical interventions and palliative therapies as well as the more traditional education, prevention, detoxification, and substitution treatments. For example, a past or present drug user on anticoagulants for past recurring thrombosis with chronic hepatic disease, excessive alcohol use, and a depressed mood are a burden for families as well as the health and social services.

Examples of comorbid conditions, often several existing at any time, are as follows.

◆ pregnancy;
◆ risk or presence of blood-borne viruses;
◆ comorbid mental health problems;
◆ vascular complications from past injecting;
◆ past medical damage caused by drug use such as thrombosis, stroke, or cardiovascular disease;
◆ degenerative conditions and cancer;
◆ drug-related death of partners or friends;
◆ associated alcohol dependency;
◆ long-standing tobacco use;
◆ the aging drug user;
◆ associated cannabis use;
◆ social isolation.

Issues related to comorbidity are noted in Table 9.3.

Table 9.2 attempts to summarize the problems associated with drug use and to put them in some sort of chronological order.

Table 9.3 Comorbidity issues

Multiple virus infections and coexisting treatments (HIV, hepatitis B and C)
Mental health problems and treatments
Compromised cardiovascular and pulmonary status
Advanced liver disease caused by hepatitis and alcohol problems
Social isolation and dependency

Other interventions which may be prioritized in the consultation include:

- education, screening, and immunizations for hepatitis B,
- increasing the drug user's awareness of new threats of hepatitis B and C,
- highlighting the actual or potential for alcohol problems,
- challenge of mobile population: need to do all possible at each encounter,
- care for the children of drug users,
- collecting and interpretation of blood-borne virus data—HIV, hepatitis B and C—and acting on audit results.

Advice and information services

Advice and information services provide factual information on drugs and drug treatment. The advice and information should be provided in an accessible and meaningful form (in terms of context, language, and comprehensibility) to the recipient. The advice and information provided can be conveyed in a variety of ways such as verbal, written, audio-visual, in person, or over the telephone. Advice and information may cover topics such as:

- potential psychological and physical implications of drug misuse;
- guidance on how to reduce or stop drug misuse safely;
- harm reduction information and guidance;
- where to get help.

Criminal justice interventions

Individuals accessing drug-treatment services may have done so as a result of engagement in a criminal justice intervention. The following describes specific criminal justice drug-treatment interventions that are provided in the community. Some of these interventions are in relation to the English criminal justice service and relevant to the laws in force in England. Scotland has similar but variable intervention and other countries may have different schemes.

Arrest Referral Schemes were introduced nationally in England and Wales from 1 April 2000. The aim of Arrest Referral Schemes is to bridge the gap between the criminal justice system and treatment services by identifying drug-user detainees and referring them into appropriate treatment shortly after arrest. Referral is not an alternative to prosecution.

Drug Treatment and Testing Orders (DTTOs) are a community sentence introduced as part of the Crime and Disorder Act 1998. Similar orders are available to the courts in Scotland and in the USA this type of sentencing has been available for some time. The order targets persistent offenders aged 16 years and over, that offend to fund serious drug dependency. The aim is to promote a reduction and/or cessation in drug use, therefore reducing drug-related crime. DTTOs run from 6 months to no more than 3 years. A DTTO can be imposed alone or alongside a Community Rehabilitation Order (which replaced Probation Orders); the duration of the 'treatment and testing period' must be specified within the order and subject to regular court review hearings. Frequent urine analysis is mandatory throughout the order. Offenders are required to give their consent before a DTTO can be made. The principle of consent is fundamental to the order due to the general medical principle that a person should not be compelled to undergo treatment without giving consent.

Drug Abstinence Orders are a community sentence introduced as part of the Crime and Disorder Act 2000. The order has similarities to DTTOs as it compels the individual serving the order to undergo regular drug testing; however, there are differences. Firstly, the aim is to be drug abstinent rather than reduce drug use, and secondly drug treatment is not a formal part of the order, although this may be undertaken voluntarily.

The research basis for treatment

Research is poor in some areas of treatment. Much is known about the efficacy of pharmacological interventions, both about its benefits and limitations. For all sorts of reasons clear research outcomes for the value of longer-term treatments are difficult to obtain. For a disorder such as addiction with many facets and spanning all sectors of society simple conclusions are not available. There are however some general observations which have been covered in this chapter.

Analysis of the outcomes of rehabilitation and self-help agency treatment

Overall the literature on the effectiveness of residential rehabilitation shows most studies to be compromised by methodological difficulties. It is difficult to study these populations and to measure hard outcomes. Generally, retention in treatment is a problem but those who stay the treatment may reduce opiate use and improve employment chances. Most studies are unclear about outcomes as individuals in treatment are mostly polydrug users and may shift from one dependency to another. The studies available also found long-term follow-up difficult so little is recorded about recovery and sustained recovery beyond 18 months or 2 years. Similarly, for self-help organizations trying to define or evaluate such organizations, which are by their very nature infinitely variable, is impossible. The essential qualities are equally problematic to categorize. Probably the most extensive contemporary work on the topic is Keith Humphreys' book called *Circles of Recovery* (Humphreys 2004). Helpfully he suggests that this group of disparate agencies are characterized by being 'voluntary associations operated by peers who share a problematic status, rely upon experiential knowledge, value reciprocal helping, do not charge fees, and include personal change among their organisational goals'.

Although it may be impossible to scientifically evaluate the overall effect of non-statutory organizations there are some general conclusions. Self-help groups seem in general to help some people reduce their dependency on illegal or addictive substances. They have an influence on the spiritual or personal identity and confidence of participants. Finally there is a significant advantage in their effect on healthcare cost savings. The advantages of organizations such as Alcoholics Anonymous and Narcotics Anonymous are disputed by few: the need for an extensive range of agencies to provide special needs for people with needs is difficult to argue against. Groups for minorities of all sorts are essential, for women with or without children, and for a host of people with personal preferences not catered for elsewhere. Requirements for agencies may be sensitive to the local needs of a particular community or geographical area and may be serviced by individuals with particular vision or groups with a commonly identified interest. They may be local, national, or international and of any size.

Conclusions

This chapter has attempted to explore the breadth of treatment services and the issues involved. Few simple conclusions are possible for the very many reasons outlined above. It is important to observe, however, that the damage caused by addiction is considerable and its impact on health and social services immeasurable. Added to these costs are the social costs of crime and the expense of the criminal justice interventions. Treatment has to be flexible and increasingly coordinated between agencies. At any point in time change is required in treatment provision and vision is essential to allow the development of suitable services for an ever-changing population of service users.

Chapter 10

Future directions

As explained in preceding chapters, it is clear that levels of drug use and drug-related problems in the UK are high by international standards. Illicit drug use has declined during recent years, but remains so widespread that it is established as normal behaviour among substantial sections of the UK population. Evidence, backed by some very weighty opinions, suggests that the eradication of illicit drug use may well be impossible. Moreover, attempts to achieve this would inevitably involve repressive policies that would be both futile and immoral. However, effective harm-minimization measures are possible and have been shown to be effective. Even so, future policies should be motivated by objective evidence of policy effectiveness and not guided solely by moral panic or draconian law enforcement. There is a serious problem when anybody daring to voice a view disputing the dictum of 'drugs are totally very bad, so don't confuse the picture by suggesting otherwise' runs the risk of being vilified by the tabloid press and some unwary politicians. Tabloid press and media hostility to any real discussion of drug issues is a destructive force that only serves to distort the debate and the issues that it involves. An example of the confusion in the policy agenda was highlighted with the recent sacking of Professor David Nutt from his chairmanship of the UK's Advisory Council on the Misuse of Drugs (ACMD). This has, sadly, served to muddy the waters even further by complicating the relationship between scientists and policy makers. There is no reason why scientific advice should always be accepted by politicians. They clearly do have the authority to consider such advice and respond to it as they see fit. Despite this, however, scientific advisers should be able to speak or write freely without running the risk of being dismissed if politicians dislike what they have to say. At present the ACMD is a damaged agency which no longer seems to have the authority and independence that it should and as a result is of questionable value. Its role and future must now be in doubt. This is not only a 'problem' for the 'drug field' in the UK but it also has important implications for all branches of scientific enquiry worldwide. This is why recent events have been given such extensive international coverage. There may be a way out of this impasse. As noted, it has already been suggested that the relationship between scientific advice and government should be guided (and protected) by the *Principles for the Treatment of Independent Scientific Advice Provided to Government* (Hood 2009b).

Distinct from the debate about national and international strategy on drug misuse are the regional and local requirements for health and care services for those requiring help for drug-related problems or treatment for a complication of drug use. In this text there have been numerous examples of the needs for treatment and rehabilitation services and an increasing demand for medical care for the severe complications of drug use. There seems an inevitability that these problems are likely to increase and that additional services will be required as well as the expansion of existing agencies. Already mental health services are being overwhelmed with serious complications of alcohol and drug taking. Ominous signs of an impending epidemic of cirrhosis and liver disease caused by alcohol and hepatitis C threaten to provide an unprecedented demand for medical expertise and hospital care and an already compromised healthcare system is facing a new level of demand from ageing drug users with cardiovascular, respiratory, and brain problems. All this comes at a time of cutbacks and constraints due to worldwide economic downturn. Never has there been a greater need for services to concentrate on the essential, the effective, and the attractive to patients' treatments.

Prevention is one of the principal pillars of drug policy in the UK and most other countries. Intuitively the most attractive and cost-effective response to the 'drug problem' is to educate and support young people in an attempt to prevent the onset of drug use. There can be little doubt that this is the ideal policy with the most attractive outcome. It has, however, been explained in this text that drug education and related mass-media campaigns have been convincingly shown not to discourage or reduce levels of drug use. This disappointing fact is not widely known (or acknowledged), even to those who are practitioners of these activities. This is one area where national drug policy could be far more evidence-based. It must be strongly recommended that public funding should no longer be wasted on something that is so clearly ineffective. Effective interventions need to be identified and supported by adequate funds on a secure basis with careful monitoring, associated research, and continued training and development for participants. Those working in other areas of treatment and social support are well aware of the need to have permanent funding, career development, and academic support as well as an evidence-based infrastructure with the confidence of the community and the clients. There are few organizations outside the generic primary care and mental health services with such a structure and these agencies struggle to cope with a difficult demand from an ever-changing population of drug and alcohol users.

The future looks far from attractive and signs of improvement either in the size of the caseload or the ability of services to respond are hard to find. Inevitably governments are going to face difficult decisions but as time goes on expenditure will continue to rise and the needs of drug users will assume a more pressing political force. As this pressure increases the best possible under-standing of the nature of drug dependence and misuse will be required and pragmatic solutions will have to be made available.

Bibliography

The following references were invaluable in the writing of this book. Many, though not all, have been cited in the text.

Abrams, M. (1959) *The teenage consumer*. London: Press Exchange.

Academy of Medical Sciences (2004a) *Calling time: The nation's drinking as a health issue*. London: Academy of Medical Sciences.

Academy of Medical Sciences (2004b) *Prime Minister's Strategy Unit report on alcohol misuse* (press release), 15 March. London: Academy of Medical Sciences.

Adamson, P. (2007) *Child poverty in perspective: An overview of child well-being in rich countries*, Innocenti Report Card, vol. 7. Florence: UNICEF Innocenti Research Centre.

Advisory Committee on Drug Dependence (1968) *Cannabis*. London: HMSO.

Advisory Council on the Misuse of Drugs (1998) *Drug misuse and the environment*. London: HMSO.

Advisory Council on the Misuse of Drugs (2000) *Reducing drug-related deaths*. London: Home Office.

Advisory Council on the Misuse of Drugs (2002) *The classification of cannabis under the Misuse of Drugs Act 1971*. London: Home Office.

Advisory Council on the Misuse of Drugs (2003) *Hidden harm: Responding to the needs of children of problem drug users main report*. London: Home Office. http://drugs. homeoffice.gov.uk/publication-search/acmd/hidden-harm

Advisory Council on the Misuse of Drugs (2004) *Pathways to problems: Hazardous use of tobacco, alcohol and other drugs by young people in the UK and its implications for policy*. London: Home Office.

Advisory Council on the Misuse of Drugs (2005) *Further consideration of the classification of cannabis under the Misuse of Drugs Act 1971*. London: Home Office.

Advisory Council on the Misuse of Drugs (2006) *Further consideration of the classification of cannabis under the Misuse of Drugs Act 1971*. London: Home Office.

Advisory Council on the Misuse of Drugs (2007) *Hidden harm: Three years on: realities, challenges and opportunities*. London: Home Office.

Advisory Council on the Misuse of Drugs (2008) *Cannabis: Classification and public health*. London: Home Office.

Advisory Council on the Misuse of Drugs (2009a) *MDMA ('ecstasy'): A review of its harms and classification under the Misuse of Drugs Act 1971*. London: Home Office.

Advisory Council on the Misuse of Drugs (2009b) *Consideration of the major cannabinoid agonists*, 16 July, http://drugs.homeoffice.gov.uk/publication-search/acmd/acmd-report-agonists?view=Binary

Afitska, N., Plant, M.A., Weir, I., Miller, P. and Plant, M.L. (2008) The relationship between teenage "binge" drinking, age of first alcohol consumption and intoxication. *Journal of Substance Use* **13**, 205–18.

Akhtar, P., Corbett, J., Currie, C. and Currie, D. (2004) *Scottish Schools Adolescent Lifestyle and Substance Use Survey (SALUS) national report.* Norwich: TSO.

Aldgate, J. and McIntosh, M. (2006) *Looking after the family: A study of children looked after in kinship care in Scotland.* Edinburgh: Social Work Inspection Agency.

Alexander, B. (2008) *The globalisation of addiction.* Oxford: Oxford University Press.

American Psychiatric Association (2000) DSM iv. Washington DC: American Psychiatric Association

American Public Health Association (2007) *Acting Surgeon General issues national call to action on underage drinking* (press release), 6 March, p. 1, http://www.apha.org/membergroups/newsletters/sectionnewsletters/alcohol/winter07/underagedrinking.htm

Amt, E. (ed.) (1993) *Women's lives in medieval Europe.* London: Routledge.

Anderson, K. and Plant, M.A. (1996) Abstaining and carousing: substance use among adolescents in the Western Isles of Scotland. *Drug and Alcohol Dependence* **41**, 198–6.

Andronik, C.M. (2007) *Wildly romantic: The English Romantic Poets: The mad, the bad and the dangerous.* New York: Henry Holt and Company.

Anonymous (2009) http://www.drugtext.org/index.php/ru/press/974-international-drugs-body-calls-for global-action-as-internet-dealing

Aquilino, W.S. and Losciuto, L.A. (1990) Effects of interview mode on self-reported drug use. *Public Opinion Quarterly* **54**, 362–95.

Ashton, H. (1994) The treatment of benzodiazepine dependence. *Addiction* **89**, 1535–41.

Ashton, M. (ed.) (1992) *The ecstasy papers: A collection of ISDD's publications on the dance drugs phenomenon.* London: Institute for the Study of Drug Dependence.

Association of Chief Police Officers (2007) *Guidance on policing cannabis.* London: Association of Chief Police Officers of England, Wales and Northern Ireland.

Asthana, A. (2005) One bar, three hours-I was sold enough drink to kill me. *The Observer* **24** October, pp. 8–9.

Austin, E.W., Chen, J.C. and Grube, J.W. (2006) How does alcohol advertising influence underage drinking? The role of desirability, identification and scepticism. *Journal of Adolescent Health* **38**, 376–84.

Babor, T., Higgins-Biddle, J.C., Saunders, J.S. and Monteiro, M. (2001) *The alcohol use disorders identification test: Guidelines for use in primary care,* 2nd edn. Geneva: World Health Organization.

Babor, T., Caetano, R., Casswell, S., Edwards, G., Giesbrecht, N., Graham, K., Grube, J., Gruenwald, P., Hill, L., Holder, H. et al. (2003) *Alcohol: No ordinary commodity.* Oxford: Oxford University Press.

Baer, J.S., Marlatt, A. and Mcmahon, R.J. (eds) (1993) *Addictive behaviors across the life span.* London: Sage.

Báez, H., Castro, M.M., Benavente, M.A., Kintz, P., Cirimele, V., Camargo, C. and Thomas, C. (2000) Drugs in prehistory: chemical analysis of ancient human hair. *Forensic Science International* **108**, 173–9.

Baggott, R. (1990) *Alcohol, politics & social policy.* Avebury: Gower Publishing Company.

Balarajant, R. and Yuen, P. (1986) British smoking and drinking habits: regional variations. *Community Medicine* **8**, 131–7.

Bancroft, A., Wilson, S., Cunningham-Burley, S. Backett-Milburn, K. and Masters, H. (2004) *Parental drug and alcohol use*. York: Joseph Rowntree Foundation.

Bandy, P. and President, P.A. (1983) Recent literature on drug abuse and prevention and mass media: focusing on youth, parents, women and elderly. *Journal of Drug Education* **13**, 255–71.

Bangert-Drowns, R. (1988) The effects of school-based substance abuse education – a meta-analysis. *Journal of Drug Education* **18**, 243–64.

Banta-Green, C., Field, J., Chiaia, A.C., Sudakin, D.L., Power, L. and de Montigny, L. (2009) The spatial epidemiology of cocaine, methamphetamine and 3,4-methylenedi-oxymethamphetamine (MDMA) use: a demonstration using a population measure of community drug load derived from municipal wastewater. *Addiction* **104**, 1874–80.

Barker, D.J.F. (1973) *Practical epidemiology*. Edinburgh: Churchill Livingstone.

Barker, W., Homel, P., Flaherty, B. and Trebilco, P. (1987) *The 1986 Survey of Drug Use by Secondary School Students in New South Wales*. Sydney: New South Wales Drug and Alcohol Authority In-House Report Series.

Barn, R. (2001) *Black youth on the margins: A research revie*. York: Joseph Rowntree Foundation.

Barnard, M. (1999) ladettes large it in Liverpool. *The Times Weekend* 18 September, p. 29.

Barnard, M.A. and Forsyth, A.J.M. (1998) Drug use among schoolchildren in rural Scotland. *Addiction Research* **6**, 431–24.

Barnard, M.A., Forsyth, A.J.M. and McKegany, N.P. (1996) Levels of drug use among a sample of Scottish schoolchildren. *Drugs: Education, Prevention and Policy* **3**, 81–89.

Barnes, G.M. (2005) Adolescent alcohol abuse and other problem behaviours: their relationships and common parental influences. *Journal of Youth and Adolescence* **13**, 329–48.

Barnes, G.M. and Farrell, M.P. (1992) Parental support and control as predictors of adolescent drinking, delinquency and related problem behaviours. *Journal of Marriage and the Family* **54**, 763–76.

Barr, A. (1995) *Drink: An informal social history*. London: Bantam.

Bashford, J., Buffin, J. and Patel, K. (2003) *The Department of Health's Black and Minority Ethnic Drug Misuse Needs Assessment Project*, Report 2: The Findings. Preston: Centre for Ethnicity and Health.

Baum, D. (1996) Smoke and mirrors. In: *The war on drugs and the politics of failure*, pp. 13–29. New York: Little Brown.

Baumrind, D. (1991) The influence of parenting style on adolescent competence and substance use. *Journal of Early Adolescence* **11**, 56–95.

BBC (2001) *BBC/ICM poll on attitudes to drug laws reported*, 6 February.

BBC (2004) *Healthy Britain survey*, 9 August.

BBC News Online (2005) *Magic mushrooms ban becomes law*, 18 July, http://news.bbc.co.uk/1/hi/uk/4691899.stm

BBC News Online (2007a) *Cameron defiant over drug claims*, 11 February, http://news.bbc.co.uk/1/hi/uk_politics/6351331.stm

BBC News online (2007b) *UK is accused of failing children*, 14 February, http://news.bbc.co.uk/1/hi/uk/6359363.stm

BBC News Online (2007c) *Top ministers admit cannabis use*, 20 July, http://news.bbc.co. uk/1/hi/uk_politics/6907040.stm

BBC News Online (2008a) *Police want cannabis reclassified*, 3 April, http://news.bbc.co. uk/1/hi/uk/7328673.stm

BBC News Online (2008b) *Taliban's $100m opium takings*, report by Kate Clark, 24 June, http://news.bbc.co.uk/1/hi/world/south_asia/7469194.stm

BBC News online (2008c) *Tough-on-drugs policy "pointless,"* 13 August. http://news.bbc. co.uk/1/hi/uk/7557708.stm

BBC News Online (2009a) *Concern over white heroin return*, 1 February, http://news.bbc. co.uk/1/hi/uk/7863352.stm

BBC News Online (2009b) *Cocaine A&E cases hit record high*, report by Jim Reed, 13 July, http://news.bbc.co.uk/newsbeat/hi/health/newsid 8147000/8147446.stm

BBC News Online (2009c) *Drug –driving campaign is launched*, 17 August, http://news.bbc. co.uk/1/hi/uk/8201407.stm

BBC News Online (2009d) *"Legal highs" set to be banned*, 25 August, http://news.bbc.co. uk/1/hi/uk/8218688.stm

BBC News Online (2010a) *Over 1,000 Britons are jailed over drugs abroad*, 3 February, http://news.bbc.co.uk/1/hi/uk/8493551.stm

BBC News Online (2010b) *Rise in cocaine use alarms UK government drug advisors*, 2 March, http://news.bbc.co.uk/1/hi/uk/8544648.stm

Bean, P. (1974) *The social control of drugs*. London: Martin Robertson.

Bean, P. (ed.) (1993) *Cocaine and crack: Supply and use*. London: Macmillan Press.

Bean, P. (2004) *Drugs and crime*. Uffculme, Devon: Willan Publishing.

Beck, F. and Legleye, S. (2003) *Drogues et adolecents. Usages de drogues et contexts d'usage entre 17 et 19 ans, évolutions récents*, ESCAPAD (2002). Paris: OFDT.

Becker, H.S. (1953–1954) Becoming a marihuana user. *American Journal of Sociology* **LIX**, 235–42.

Beckley Foundation (2005) *Facing the future: The challenge for national & international drug policy*. Oxford: Beckley Foundation.

Bell, J.E., and Zador, D. (2000) A risk-benefit analysis of methadone maintenance treatment. *Drug Safety* **22**, 179–90.

Bell, J.E., Arango, C.-J., Robertson, J.R., Brettle, R.P., Leen, C. and Simmonds, P. (2002) HIV and drug misuse in the Edinburgh cohort. *Journal of Acquired Immune Deficiency Syndromes* **31**, 35–42.

Bellis, M.A., Weild, A.W., Beeching, N.J., Mutton, K. and Syed, Q. (1997) Prevalence of HIV and injecting drug use in men entering Liverpool Prison, England. *British Medical Journal* **315**, 30–1.

Bellis, M.A., Beynon, C., Millar, T., Ashton, J.R., Djuretic, T. and Taylor, A. (2001) Unexplained illness and deaths among injecting drug users in England: a case control study using Regional Drug Misuse Databases. *Journal of Epidemiology and Community Health* **55**, 843–4.

Bellis, M.A., Hennell, T., Lushey, C., Hughes, K., Tocque, K. and Ashton, J.R. (2007) Elvis to Eminem: quantifying the price of fame through early mortality of European and North American rock and pop stars. *Journal of Epidemiology and Community Health* **61**, 896–901.

Berridge, V. (1989) Historical issues. In: MacGregor, S. (ed), *Drugs and British society*. London: Tavistock/Routledge.

Berridge, V. (1999) *Opium and the people. Opiate use and drug control policy in nineteenth and early twentieth century England*. London: Free Association Books.

Bestic, A. (1966) *Turn me on man*. London: Tandem.

Betty Ford Institute Panel (2009) What is recovery. *Mental Health and Substance Use* **2**, 259–62.

Bewley, T.H. (1965) Heroin Addiction in the United Kingdom (1954-1964). *British Medical Journal* **2**, 1284–6.

Bewley, T.H. (1966) Recent changes in the pattern of drug abuse in the United Kingdom. *Bulletin of Narcotics* **28**, 1–13.

Binnie, H.L. and Murdock, G. (1969) *Attitudes to drugs and drugtakers of students at the university and colleges of higher education in an English midland city*, University of Leicester, Vaughan Papers, No 14. Oxford: Oxford University Press.

Bird, S.M. (2007) Compulsory drugs testing in the British Army: assessing the data. *RUSI Journal* **152**, 54–9.

Bird, J. (2008) *Afghanistan diary*, http://news.bbc.co.uk/1/hi/scotland/7582380.stm

Birtalan, D. (2005) *Parental guidance regarding alcohol is the most effective influence on student drinking*, report related to Tufts Alcohol and Drug Use Survey, http://list.web.net/archives/apolnet-!/2005-March/000202.html

Bjarnason, T. (1995) Administration mode bias in a school survey on alcohol, tobacco and illicit drug use. *Addiction* **90**, 555–9.

Bjarnason, T. (2009) Anomie among European adolescents: conceptual and empirical clarification of a multilevel sociological concept. *Sociological Forum* **24**, 135–61.

Black, S. and Casswell, S. (1993) *Drugs in New Zealand society- a survey 1990*. Auckland: Alcohol and Public Health Research Unit, University of Auckland.

Blackman, S. (2004) *Chilling out: The cultural politics of substance consumption, youth and drug policy*. Maidenhead: Open University Press.

Blane, D. (1996) Collecting retrospective data: Development of a reliable method and a pilot study of its use. *Social Science and Medicine* **42**, 751–7.

Bloomfield, K., Allamani, A., Beck, F., Bergmark, K., Csemy, L., Eisenbach-Stangl, E., Elekes, Z., Gmel, G., Kerr Correa, F., Knibbe, R. et al. (2005) *Gender, culture & alcohol-related problems: A multi-national study; project final report*. Berlin: Charité Universitätsmedizin.

BMRB International Ltd (1995) *National drugs campaign report*. London: BMRB International Ltd.

Boardman, J.D., Finch, B.K., Ellison, C.G., Williams, D.R. and Jackson, J.S. (2001) Neighbourhood disadvantages, stress and drug use among adults. *Journal of Health and Social Behaviour* **42**, 151–65.

Bonnie, R.J. and O'Connell, M.E. (eds) (2003) *Reducing underage drinking*. Washington DC: The National Academies Press.

Booth, C. (1902) *Life and labour of the people in London*. London: Macmillan and Co.

Borawski, E., Ievers-Landis, C., Lovegreen, L. and Trapl, E. (2003) Parental monitoring, negotiated unsupervised time, and parental trust: the role of perceived parenting practices in adolescent health risk behaviors. *Journal of Adolescent Health* **33**, 60–70.

Boseley, S. (2009) Drink and drugs a leading cause of youth deaths. *The Guardian* 11 September, p. 7.

Bowden, M. (2001) *Killing Pablo.* New York: Atlantic Books.

Boyd, G.M., Howard, J. and Zucker, R.A. (eds) (1995) *Alcohol problems among adolescents.* Hove: Lawrence Erlbaum Associates.

Boys, A., Farrell, M., Bebbington, P., Brugha, T., Coid, J., Jenkins, R., Lewis, G., Marsden, J., Meltzer, H., Singleton, N. and Taylor, C. (2002) Drug use and initiation in prison: results from a national prison survey in England and Wales. *Addiction* **97**, 1551–60.

Bradshaw, S. (1972) *Drug misuse and the law.* London: McMillan.

Bradshaw, S. and Richardson. D. (2009) *An index of child wellbeing in Europe.* York: Social Policy Research Unit. http://php.york.ac.uk/inst/spru/pubs/1175/

Brain Reports -See Interdepartmental Committee on Drug Addiction.

Brake, M. (1985) *Comparative youth culture.* London: Routledge and Kegan Paul.

British Medical Association (1997) *Therapeutic uses of cannabis.* Amsterdam: Harwood Academic.

British Medical Association (2008) *Alcohol misuse: Tackling the UK epidemic.* London: British Medical Association.

British Medical Association and Royal Pharmaceutical Society of Great Britain (2009) *British national formulary,* 57th edn. London: British Medical Association and Royal Pharmaceutical Society of Great Britain.

Brown, C. and Lawton, J. (1988) *Illicit drug use in Portsmouth and Havant.* London: Policy Studies Institute.

Brown, J.H. (2001) Youth, drugs and resilience education. *Journal of Drug Education* **31**, 83–122.

Brown, J. and Langton, D. (2007) Legalise all drugs: chief constable demands end to "immoral laws". *The Independent* 15 October, http://www.independent.co.uk/news/uk/politics/legalise-all-drugs-chief-constable-demands-end-to-immoral-laws-396884.html

Brown, M. and Bolling, K. (2007) *Drugs misuse in Scotland: Findings from the 2006 Scottish Crime and Victimisation Survey.* Edinburgh: Scottish Government Social Research.

Brown, W.C. (2010) Nutt damage. *Lancet* **375**, 724.

Bruner, T.F. (1973) Marijuana in Ancient Greece and Rome? The Literary Evidence. *Bulletin of the History of Medicine* **47**, 344–55.

Bruun, K. (1986) Everything was medicine in the beginning. *Drinking and Drug Practices Surveyor* **21**, 3–5.

Bruun, K., Edwards, G., Lumio, M., Mäkelä, K., Pan, L., Popham R., Room, R., Schmidt, W., Skog, Ø-J., Sulkunen, P. and Sterberg, E. (1975a) *Alcohol control policies in public health perspective.* Helsinki: Finnish Foundation for Alcohol Studies.

Bruun, K., Pan, L. and Rexed, I. (1975b) The gentleman's club. In: *International control of drugs & alcohol.* Chicago: University of Chicago Press.

Bryan, J. (2009) The discovery of benzodiazepines and the adverse publicity that followed. *Pharmaceutical Journal* **283**, 305–6.

Buchan, T. (2002) *A cultural and spatial analysis of adolescent substance misuse in rural Wales: final report,* research report 11. Powys: Institute of Rural Health.

Budd, J. and Robertson, J.R. (2005) Hepatitis C and general practice: the crucial role of primary care in stemming the epidemic. *British Journal of General Practice* **55**, 259–60.

Budd, J., Copeland, L., Elton, R.A. and Robertson, J.R. (2002) Hepatitis C infections in a cohort of injecting drug users - past and present risk factors and the implications for educational and clinical management. *The European Journal of General Practice* **8**, 95–100.

Budd, T. (2003) *Alcohol-related assault: Findings from the British Crime Survey*, online report 35/03. London: Home Office.

Bull, M. (2008) *Governing the heroin trade*. Abingdon: Ashgate.

Burns, L., Flaherty, B., Ireland, S. and Frances, M. (1995) Policing pubs: what happens to crime? *Drug and Alcohol Review* **14**, 369–75.

Cabinet Office Prime Minister's Strategy Unit (2003) *Alcohol project: Interim analytic report*. London: Cabinet Office.

Cabinet Office Prime Minister's Strategy Unit (2004) *Alcohol harm reduction strategy for England*. London: Cabinet Office.

Caetano, R. (2001) Non-response in alcohol and drug surveys: a research topic in need of further attention. *Addiction* **96**, 1541–5.

Calder, I.M. and Ramsay, J. (1987) A survey of cannabis use in offshore rig workers. *British Journal of Addiction* **82**, 159–61.

Campbell, D. (2009a) International drugs body calls for global action as internet dealing rises to "alarming" levels. *The Guardian* 19 February, p. 18.

Campbell, D. (2009b) Heavy drinkers not getting enough NHS help, report says. *The Guardian* 30 July, p. 11.

Campbell, D. (2010) Teenagers damaged by legal "cocaine." *The Observer* 17 January, p. 19.

Campbell, D. and Hirsch, A. (2009) Rift with EU as US sticks to Bush line on "war on drugs". *The Guardian* 3 February, p. 18.

Canning, U., Millward, L., Raj, T. and Warm, D. (2004) *Drug use prevention among young people: A review of reviews: Evidence briefing*. London: Health Development Agency.

Casey, C. (1994) Supergrass. *Police Review*, 4 March, 16–7.

Carrell, S. (2010) Nationwide alert after six addicts die from anthrax-tainted heroin. *The Guardian* 8 January, p. 11.

Carter, H. (2004) Police force lottery over drug law. *The Guardian* 23 January, p. 1.

Cavan, S. (1966) *Liquor license: An ethnography of bar behavior*. Chicago: Aldine.

Central Policy Review Staff (1979) *Alcohol policies in the United Kingdom*. Stockholm: Sociologiska Institutionen, Stockholms Universitat (printed in 1982).

Chambers, G. and Tombs, J. (1984) *The British Crime Survey: Scotland*. London: HMSO.

Chatterton, P. and Holland, R. (2003) *Urban nightscapes: Youth cultures, pleasure spaces and corporate power*. London: Routledge.

Coats, J. (2006) *No big deal: A guide to recovery from addictions*. Aldborough, Suffolk: Sow's Ear Press.

Cocket, R. (1971) *Drug abuse and personality in young offenders*. London: Butterworths.

Cohen, R. (1965) *Drugs of hallucination*. London: Secker and Warburg.

Cohen, S. (ed.) (1971) *Images of deviance*. Harmondsworth: Penguin.

Cohen, S. (1972) *Folk devils and moral panics*. London: MacGibbon and Kee.

Coleman, J. and Hagell, A. (eds) (2007) *Adolescence, risk and resilience: against the odds*. Chichester: Wiley.

Collaboration TATC (2008) Life expectancy of individuals on combination antiretroviral therapy in high income countries: a collaborative analysis of 14 cohort studies. *Lancet* **372**, 272–9.

Collins, J.J. Jr (ed.) (1982) *Drinking and crime.* London: Tavistock.

Colorado Alcohol and Drug Abuse Division (1990) *Analysis of selected alcohol and drug related risk factors for the 634 countries and statewide average, 1986-1990.* Denver, CO: Colorado Alcohol and Drug Abuse Division.

Comeau, N., Stewart, S.H. and Loba, P. (2001) The relations of trait anxiety, anxiety sensitivity, and sensation seeking to adolescents' motivations for alcohol, cigarette, and marijuana use. *Addictive Behaviors* **26**, 803–25.

Committee on Safety of Medicines (1988) Benzodiazepines, dependence and withdrawal symptoms. *Current Problems* **21**, 1–?

Connell, D., Tumer, R. and Mason, E. (1985) Summary of finding of the School Health Education evaluation: health promotion effectiveness, implementation, and costs. *Journal of School Health* **55**, 316–21.

Connell, P.H. (1964) Amphetamine misuse. *British Journal of Addiction* **60**, 9–27.

Consensus Conference (1992) Guidelines for the management of patients with generalised anxiety. *Psychiatric Bulletin* **16**, 560–5.

Coomber, R. (1997a) How often does the adulteration/dilution of heroin actually occur: an analysis of 228 "street" samples across the UK (1995-1996) and discussion of monitoring policy. *International Journal of Drug Policy* **8**, 178–86.

Coomber, R. (1997b) Vim in the veins - fantasy or fact: the adulteration of illicit drugs. *Addiction Research* **5**, 195–212.

Coomber, R. (1997c) The adulteration of drugs: what dealers do, what dealers think. *Addiction Research* **5**, 297–306.

Coomber, R. (1997d) Adulteration of drugs: the discovery of a myth. *Contemporary Drug Problems* **24**, 239–71.

Coomber, R. (1999) Cutting the crap: the reality of drug adulteration. *Druglink* July/ August **14**, 19–21.

Copeland, L., Budd, J., Elton, R.A. and Robertson J.R. (2004) The changing patterns in causes of death in a cohort of injecting drug users 1980 – 2001. *Archives of Internal Medicine* **164**, 1214–20.

Corkery, J. (2002) *Drug seizure and offender statistics: United Kingdom 2000.* London: Home Office.

Corkery, J. (2008) UK drug-related mortality- issues in definition and classification. *Drugs and Alcohol Today* **8**, 17–25.

Coughlin, C. (2008) Afghanistan swaps heroin for wheat, Telegraph.co.uk, 8 April, http://blogs.telegraph.co.uk/politics/threelinewhip/april08/afghanistanswapsheroinforwheat.htm

Courtwright, D.T. (1982) *Dark paradise,* Cambridge, MA: Harvard University Press.

Courtwright, D.T. (2001) *Forces of habit: Drugs and the making of the modern world.* Cambridge, MA: Harvard University Press.

Crawford, A. (1987) Bias in a survey of drinking habits. *Alcohol and Alcoholism* **22**, 167–79.

Crawford, A. (2008) Data laws hamper MoD prison study. *BBC News Online* 22 October, http://news.bbc.co.uk/1/hi/uk/7682964.stm

Crawford, A., Plant, M.A., Kreitman, N. and Latcham, R.W. (1984) Myth Uncovered? II Population Surveys. *British Medical Journal* **289**, 1343–5.

Crombie, I., Irvine, L., Elliott, L. and Wallace, H. (2005) *Public health policy on alcohol*. Dundee: University of Dundee/NHS Health Scotland.

Crome, I., Ghodse, H., Gilvarry, E. and McArdle, P. (2003) *Young people and substance misuse*. London: Gaskell.

Crowley, A. (1922) *Diary of a drug fiend*. London: Collins.

Crowley, J.T., Macdonald, M.J., Whitmore, E.A. and Mikulich, S.K. (1998) Cannabis dependence, withdrawal, and reinforcing effects among adolescents with conduct symptoms and substance use disorders. *Drug and Alcohol Dependence* **50**, 27–37.

Csete, J., Gathumbi, A., Wolfe, D. and Cohen, J. (2009) Lives to save: PEPFAR, HIV, and injecting drug use in Africa. *Lancet* **373**, 2006–7.

Cull, W.L., O'Connor, K.G., Sharp, S. and Tang, S-f.S. (2005) Response rates and response bias for 50 surveys of pediatricians. *Health Services Research* **40**, 213–26.

Currie, C., Nic Gabhainn, S., Godeau, E., Roberts, C., Smith, R., Currie, D., Picket, W., Richter, M., Morgan, A. and Barnekow, V. (eds) (2008) *Inequalities in young people's health: International report from the HBSC 2006/06 survey*, WHO Policy Series: Health Policy for Children and Adolescents, issue 5. Copenhagen: WHO Regional Office for Europe. http://www.euro.who.int/Document/E91416_Ch2_4.pdf

Daily Mail (2007) The most idiotic police chief in Britain. *Daily Mail* January, p. 1.

Daily Mail Scotland (2006) Scottish Police in call to legalise all drugs. *Daily Mail Scotland* 13 April, p. 1.

Davenport, J. (2004) MET chief: cannabis law is in a muddle. *Evening Standard* 15 January, p. 1.

Davenport-Hines, R. (2004) *The pursuit of oblivion: A global history of narcotics*. New York: W.W. Norton & Company.

Dawtry, F. (ed.) (1968) *Social problems of drug abuse*. London: Butterworths.

De Alarcon, R. (1969) The spread of heroin abuse in a community. *Bulletin of Narcotics* **21**, 17–22.

De Alarcon, R. and Rathod, N.H. (1968) Prevalence and early detection of heroin abuse. *British Medical Journal* 2(5604): 549–53.

Dean, A. (1990) Culture and community: drink and soft drugs in Hebridean youth culture. *Sociology Review* **38**, 517–65.

Dean, A. (1995) Space and substance misuse in rural communities. *International Journal of Sociology and Social Policy* **15**, 132–55.

Dean, A. (2002) History, culture and substance use in a rural Scottish community. *Substance Use and Misuse* **37**, 749–65.

Deedes, W. (1970) *The drugs epidemic*. London: Tom Stacey.

Demetrovics, Z., Fountain, J. and Kraus, L. (eds) (2009) *Old and new policies, theories, research methods and drug users across Europe*. Lengerich: Pabst Science.

Dennis, M.L., Foss, M.A. and Scott, C.K. (2007) An eight-year perspective on the relationship between the duration of abstinence and other aspects of recovery. *Evaluation Review* **31**, 585–612.

Department of Health (1984) *Guidelines of good clinical practice in the treatment of drug misuse*. London: Department of Health.

Department of Health (1998) *Review of research into the effects of cannabis.* London: House of Lords Library.

Department of Health (2004) *Benzodiazepines warning,* Chief Medical Officer's Update 37, Patient Safety, January. London: Department of Health.

Department of Health (2007) *Drug misuse and dependence: UK guidelines on clinical management.* London: Department of Health.

Department of Health/Office for National Statistics (2002) *Statistics on Young People and Drug Misuse: England, 2000 and 2001,* bulletin 2002/15. London: Department of Health/Office for National Statistics.

Department of Health, Social Services and Public Safety (2000) *Strategy for reducing alcohol related harm.* Belfast: Department of Health, Social Services and Public Safety.

Department of Health, Social Services and Public Safety (2001) *Model for the joint implementation of the drug & alcohol strategies.* Belfast: Department of Health, Social Services and Public Safety.

Department of Health, Social Services and Public Safety (2006) *New strategic direction for alcohol and drugs (2006-2011).* Belfast: Department of Health, Social Services and Public Safety.

De Quincey, T. (reprinted 1995) *Confessions of an opium eater.* New York: Dover Publications (first published in the *London Magazine,* 1821).

Des Jarlais, D., Friedman, S., Friedmann, P., Wenston, J., Sotheran, J., Choopanya, K., Vanichseni, S., Raktham, S., Goldberg, D. and Frischer, M. (1995) HIV/AIDS-related behavior change among injecting drug users in different national settings. *AIDS* **9**, 611–18.

Di Clemente, R.J., Hansen, W.B. and Ponton, P.E. (1996) *Handbook of adolescent health risk behavior: Issues in clinical child psychology.* New York: Plenum.

Di Forti, M., Morgan, C., Dazzan, P., Pariante, C., Mondelli, V., Reis Marques, T., Handley, R., Luzi, S., Russo, M., Paperelli, A. et al. (2009) High-potency cannabis and the risk of psychosis. *British Journal of Psychiatry* **195**, 488–91.

Dillman, D.A. (2000) Introduction to tailored design. In: Dillman, D.A. (ed.), *Mail and internet surveys: The tailored design method,* pp. 3–31. New York: Wiley.

Doll. R. and Bradford Hill, A. (1954) The mortality of doctors in relation to their smoking habits: a preliminary report. *British Medical Journal* **1**, 1451–5.

Donnermeyer, J.F. (1993) Rural youth usage of alcohol, marihuana and "hard" drugs. *International Journal of the Addictions* **28**, 249–55.

D'Orban, P.T. (2006) Heroin dependency and delinquency in women- a study of heroin addicts in Holloway Prison. *Addiction* **65**, 65–78.

Dorling, D., Ballas, D., Fahmy, E., David, D. and Lupton, R., Rigby, J., Thomas, B. and Wheeler, B (2007) *Poverty, wealth and place in Britain 1968 to 2005.* Bristol: University of Bristol, The Policy Press.

Dorn, N. (1980) There ought to be law. *British Journal of Addiction* **75**, 73–9.

Dorn, N and South, N. (eds) (1998) *A land fit for heroin.* Aldershot: Gower.

Doward, J. and Shah, O. (2009) There are many drugs that help people get out of their minds yet stay within the law- they are called "legal highs." *The Observer* 26 April, pp. 22–3.

Drug and Alcohol Findings (2009) English National Evaluation fails to support drug education programme, http://findings.org.uk/count/downloads/download.php?file=Blueprint_1.txt

Drug and Therapeutics Bulletin (1990) The treatment of insomnia. *Drug and Therapeutics Bulletin* **28**, 97–9.

DrugScope (2004) Cannabis, online drug information, 23 January, ww.drugscope.org.uk

DrugScope (2008) How many people die from drugs?, http://www.drugscope.org.uk/resources/faqs/faqpages/how-many-people-use-drugs.htm

DrugScope (2009a) *DrugScope Street Drug Trends Survey 2009: Falling illegal drug purity 'accelerates trend' in users combining different drugs.* London: DrugScope, http://www.drugscope.org.uk/ourwork/pressoffice/pressreleases/Street_drug_trends_2009.htm

DrugScope (2009b) *Closer than you think: One in five adults knows someone with experience of drug addiction* (press release), 9 July, http://www.drugscope.org.uk/ourwork/pressoffice/pressreleases/ICM_poll_results.htm

DrugScope (2009c) *DrugScope welcomes ACMD recommendation that 'spice' products should be made illegal*, 12 August, http://www.drugscope.org.uk/ourwork/pressoffice/pressreleases/ACMD_Spice.htm

DrugScope (2010a) *Young people's drug and alcohol treatment at the crossroads. What it's for, where it's at and how to make it even better.* London: DrugScope.

DrugScope (2010b) *Drugs and Crime.* London: DrugScope, http://www.drugscope.org.uk/resources/mediaguide/crime

DrugScope (2010c) *The Misuse of Drugs Act 1971.* London: DrugScope, http://www.drugscope.org.uk/resources/drugsearch/drugsearchpages/laws

Dubow, E.F., Boxer, P. and Huesman, L.R. (2008) Childhood and adolescent predictors of early and middle adulthood alcohol use and problem drinking; the Columbia County longitudinal study. *Addiction* **103**, 36–47.

Duncan, T.E., Tildesley, E., Duncan, S.C. and Hops, H. (1995) The consistency of family and peer influences on the development of substance use in adolescence. *Addiction* **90**, 1647–60.

Drury, I. (2008) Legalising drugs would cause less harm AND cut crime, says former senior civil servant. *Daily Mail* 13 August, http://www.dailymail.co.uk/news/article-1044494/Legalising-drugs-cause-harm-AND-cut-crime-says-senior-civil-servant.html

Eaton, G., Morleo, M., Lodwick, A., Bellis, M.A. and McVeigh, J. (2005) *United Kingdom drug situation: Annual Report to the European Monitoring Centre for Drugs and Drug Addiction (EMCDDA).* London: Department of Health.

Edwards, G. (2005) *Matters of substance: Drugs — and why everyone's a user.* New York: Thomas Dunne Books.

Edwards, G. and Busch, C. (eds.) (1981) *Drug problems in Britain*, pp. 245–80. London: Academic Press.

Edwards, G., Anderson, P., Babor, T., Casswell, S., Ferrence, R., Giesbrecht, N., Godfrey, C., Holder, H., Lemmens, P., Mäkelä, K. et al. (1995) *Alcohol policy and the public good.* Oxford: Oxford University Press.

Elkind, D. (1984) Teenage thinking: implications for health care. *Paediatric Nursing* **10**, 383–5.

Elliot, J. (1995) Drug prevention placebo: how DARE wastes time, money, and police. *Reason* March, 14–21.

EMCDDA (European Monitoring Centre for Drugs and Drug Addiction) (2006) *Annual Report 2006: The state of the drugs problem in Europe.* Luxembourg: Office for Official Publications of the European Communities.

EMCDDA (European Monitoring Centre for Drugs and Drug Addiction) (2008) *Annual Report 2008: The state of the drugs problem in Europe.* Luxembourg: Office for Official Publications of the European Communities. http://www.drugsandalcohol.ie/11593/1/ EMCDDA_Annual_report_2008.pdf

EMCDDA (European Monitoring Centre for Drugs and Drug Addiction) (2009a) *The EU Drugs Action Plan (2005-2008).* http://www.emcdda.europa.eu/html.cfm/index10360-EN.html

EMCDDA (European Monitoring Centre for Drugs and Drug Addiction) (2009b) *Action on new drugs briefing paper: Understanding the 'spice' phenomenon,* a report from an EMCDDA expert meeting, 6 March 2009, Lisbon. http://www.emcdda.europa.eu/ drug-situation/new-drugs.

Engels, R.C.M.E. and Bot, T. (2001) Influences of risk factors on the quality of peer relations in adolescence. *Journal of Youth and Adolescence* **60**, 99–107.

Engels, R.C.M.E., De Leeuw, R.N.H., Poelen, E.A.P., Van Der Vorst, H., Van Der Zwaluw, C.S. and Van Leeuwe, J.F.W. (2007) The impact of parents on adolescent drinking and friendship selection processes. In: Järvinen, M. and Room, R. (eds), *Youth drinking cultures: European experiences,* pp. 101–18. Aldershot: Ashgate.

Englund, M.M., Egeland, B., Olivia, E.M. and Collins, W.A. (2008) Childhood and adult predictors of heavy drinking and alcohol use in early adulthood: a longitudinal developmental analysis. *Addiction* **103**, 23–35.

Ennett, S.T., Bauman, K.E., Foshee, V.A., Pemberton, M. and Hicks, K.A. (2001) Parent-child communication about adolescent tobacco and alcohol use: what do parents say and does it affect youth behaviour? *Journal of Marriage and the Family* **63**, 48–62.

Erickson, P.G., Riley, D.M. and Cheung, Y.W. (eds) (1997) *Harm Reduction: A new direction for drug policies and programs.* Toronto: University of Toronto Press.

Escobar, R. (2009) *Escobar.* London: Hodder and Stoughton.

Escohatado, A. (1999) *A brief history of drugs: From the stone age to the stoned age.* Rochester, VT: Park Street Press.

Eyle, A. (2001–2002) Drug education- Where do we go from here? *The Reconsider Quarterly* **1**, 1.

Fagan, J. (1993) Set and setting revisited: influences of alcohol and illicit drugs on the social context of violent events. In: Martin, S.E. (ed.), *Alcohol and interpersonal violence: Fostering multidisciplinary perspectives,* pp. 160–92. Rockville, MD: National Institute of Health.

Farrell, M., Boys, A., Bebbington, P., Brugha, T., Coid, J., Jenkins, R., Lewis, G., Meltzer, H., Marsden, J., Singleton, N. and Taylor, C. (2002) Psychosis and drug dependence: Results from a national survey of prisoners. *British Journal of Psychiatry* **181**, 393–8.

Ferguson, D.M., Horwood, L. and Swain-Campbell, N. (2002) Cannabis use and psychosocial adjustment in adolescence and young adulthood. *Addiction* **97**, 1123–35.

File, S.E. and Baldwin, H.A. (1989) Changes in anxiety in rats tolerant to, and withdrawn from, benzodiazepines: behavioural and biochemical studies. In: Tyrer, P. (ed.), *The psychopharmacology of anxiety*, pp. 28–51. Oxford: Oxford University Press.

Fillmore, K. (1988) *Alcohol across the life course: A critical review of seventy years of international research.* Toronto: Addiction Research Foundation.

Fischer, B., Kendall, P., Rehm, J. and Room, R. (1997) Charting WHO – goals for licit and illicit drugs for the year 2000: Are we "on track"? *Public Health* **111**, 271–5.

Fitzpatrick, S.M., Kaye, Q., Feathers, J., Pavia, J.A. and Marsaglia, K.M. (2009) Evidence for inter-island transport of heirlooms: luminescence dating and petrographic analysis of ceramic inhaling bowls from Carriacou, West Indies. *Journal of Archaeological Science* **36**, 596.

Ford, R. (2009) Number of military veterans in jail "has more than doubled in six years. *The Times* 25 September, p. 1, http://www.timesonline.co.uk/tol/news/uk/crime/article6848238.ece

Forensic Science Service (1996) *Drug abuse trends, Microgram Bulletin* 111 January–March. Aldermaston: Drugs Intelligence Laboratory, The Forensic Science Service.

Foresight (2007) *Drugs futures 2025?* Foresight Drug Science, Addiction & Drugs Project. London: Office of Science and Technology. http://www.foresight.gov.uk/Previous_Projects/Brain_Science_Addicon_and_Drugs/Reports_and_Publications/DrugsFutures2025/DTI-Overview.pdf

Forsyth, A. and Barnard, M. (1999) Contrasting levels of adolescent drug use between adjacent urban and rural communities in Scotland. *Addiction* **11**, 1707–18.

Foxcroft, D.R., Lister-Sharp, D. and Lowe, G. (1997) Alcohol misuse prevention for young people: A systematic review reveals methodological concerns and lack of reliable evidence of effectiveness. *Addiction* **92**, 531–7.

Foxcroft , D., Ireland, D., Lister-Sharp, D.J. and Breen, R. (2003) Longer-term primary prevention for alcohol misuse in young people: a systematic review. *Addiction* **98**, 397–411.

French, R.V. (1890) *Nineteen centuries of drink in England.* London: National Temperance Publication Depot.

Fuller, E. (ed.) (2008) *Drug use, smoking and drinking among young people in England in 2007.* London: Health and Social Care Information Centre.

Fuller, E. (ed.) (2009a) *Drug use, smoking and drinking among young people in England in 2008.* London: Health and Social Care Information Centre. http://www.ic.nhs.uk/webfiles/publications/sdd08fullreport/SDD_England_2008_full_report.pdf

Fuller, E. (2009b) *Trends in drinking, smoking and drug use amongst school pupils in England,* presentation at 66th Alcohol Problems Research Symposium, Kendal, 18 March.

Furst, P.T. (ed.) (1972) *Flesh of the gods: The ritual use of hallucinogens.* New York: Waveland Press.

Gabe, J. (1991) Personal troubles and public issues: the sociology of long-term tranquilliser use. In J. Gabe (ed.), *Understanding tranquilliser use: the role of the social sciences,* pp. 31–47. London: Tavistock/Routledge.

Galai, N., Safaeien, M., Vlahov, D., Bolotin, A. and Celentano, D.D. (2003) Longitudinal patterns of drug injection behaviour in the ALIVE study cohort, 1988-2000: description and determinants. *American Journal of Epidemiology* **158**, 695–704.

Garretsen, H. (2009) *The end of an era: Reflections on Dutch policies towards alcohol and drugs*, paper presented at 35th Alcohol Epidemiology Symposium of the Kettil Bruun Society, 3 June.

General Register Office for Scotland (2008) *Drug-related deaths in Scotland in 2007*. Edinburgh: General Register Office for Scotland, http://www.gro-scotland.gov.uk/files1/stats/drug-related-deaths-in-scotland 2007/drug-related-deaths-in-scotland-2007.pdf

General Register Office for Scotland (2009) *Drug-related deaths in Scotland in 2008*. Edinburgh: General Register Office for Scotland, http://www.gro-scotland.gov.uk/files2/stats/drug-related-deaths/drug-related-deaths-in-scotland-in-2008.pdf

Gfroerer, J., Lessler, J. and Parsley, T. (1997) Studies of non-response and measurement error in the national household survey on drug abuse. In: Harrison, A. and Hughes, A. (eds), *The validity of self- reported drug use: Improving the accuracy of survey estimates*, NIDA Research Monograph no. 167, p. 167. Washington DC: DHHS-NIDA.

Ghodse, H. (ed.) (2008) *International drug control into the 21st century*. Abingdon: Ashgate.

Gibbons, E. (2001) *All beer and skittles: A short history of inns and taverns*. London: The National Trust.

Gill, A.A. (2005) *The angry island*. London: Orion.

Glantz, M.D. and Leshner, A.I. (2000) Drug abuse and developmental psychopathology. *Development and Psychopathology* **12**, 795–814.

Gliksman, L. and Smythe, M. (1990) A review of school-based drug education programs: do we expect too much? In: Engs, R. (ed.), *Controversies in the addiction's field*, pp. 175–83. Kendal-Hunt: Dubuque.

Goddard, E. (2006) *Smoking and drinking among adults, 2006 (General Household Survey)*. London: Office for National Statistics.

Goddard, E. and Higgins, V. (1999) *Smoking, drinking and drug use among young teenagers in 1998*. London: The Stationery Office.

Goddard, E., Plant, M.A. Plant, M.L., Davidson, I. and Garretsen, H. (2000) Drinking patterns. In: Plant, M.A. and Cameron, I. (eds), *The alcohol report*, pp. 56–78. London: Free Association Books.

Godfrey, C. (1997) Can tax be used to minimise harm? A health economist's perspective. In: Plant, M.A., Single, E. and Stockwell, T. (eds), *Alcohol: Minimising the harm: What works?*, pp. 29–42. London: Free Association Books.

Godfrey, C., Eaton, G., McDougall, C. and Culyer, A. (2002) *The economic and social costs of class a drug use in England and Wales, 2000*, Home Office Research Study 249. London: Home Office.

Goldacre, B. (2009) Cocaine study that got up the nose of the US. *The Guardian* 13 June, p. 8.

Goode, E. (1969a) Multiple drug use amongst marijuana smokers. *Social Problems* **17**, 54–62.

Goode, E. (1969b) *Marihuana*. New York: Atherton Press.

Goode, E. (1970) *The marihuana smokers*. New York: Basic Books.

Goode, E. (1972) *Drugs in American society*. New York: Alfred A. Knopf.

Goodstadt, M. (1986) School-based drug education in North America: What is wrong? What can be done? *Journal of School Health* **56**, 278–81.

Goodstadt, M. (1989) Drug education: the prevention issues. *Journal of Drug Education* **19**, 197–208.

Goossens, L., Beyers, W., Emmen, M. and van Aken, M. (2002) The imaginary audience and Personal Fable: factor analyses and concurrent validity of the "new look" measures. *Journal of Research on Adolescence* **12**, 193–215.

Gossop, M. (2007) *Living with drugs.* Abingdon: Ashgate.

Gottleib, A. (2006) *Legal highs: A concise encyclopedia of legal herbs and chemicals with psychoactive properties.* Berkley: Ronin.

Graham, K. and Homel, R. (1997) Creating safer bars. In: Plant, M.A., Single, E. and Stockwell, T. (eds), *Alcohol: Minimising the harm: What works?*, pp. 171–92. London: Free Association Books.

Graham, K., LaRoque, L., Yetman, R., Ross, T.J. and Guistra, E. (1980) Aggression and barroom environments. *Journal of studies on Alcohol* **41**, 277–92.

Grant, B.F. and Dawson, D.A. (1997) Age at onset of alcohol use and its association with DSM-IV alcohol abuse and dependence: results from the national longitudinal alcohol epidemiologic survey. *Journal of Substance Abuse* **9**, 103–10.

Gray, C. (1995) Cannabis: the therapeutic potential. *Pharmacological Journal* **254**, 771–71.

Gray, M. (1998) *Drug crazy: How we got into this mess and how we can get out.* New York: Random House.

Green, J. and Plant, M.A. (2007) Bad bars: a review of risk factors. *Journal of Substance Use* **12**, 157–89.

Grice, A. (2004) We will reverse "absurd" reform of cannabis law, says Howard. *The Independent* 22 January, p. 1.

Griffiths, C., Romeri, E., Brock, A. and Morgan, O. (2008) Geographical variations in deaths related to substance misuse in England and Wales 1993-2006. *Health Statistics Quarterly* **39**, 14–21.

Gunn, J., Maden, A. and Swinton, M. (1991) Treatment needs of prisoners with psychiatric disorders. *British Medical Journal* **303**, 338–41.

Hackwood, F. (1910) *Inns, ales and drinking customs of Old England.* Simsbury, CT: Bracken Books (reprinted in 1985).

Hadfield, P (ed.) (2009) *Nightlife and crime.* Oxford: Oxford University Press.

Hadfield, P. and Measham, F. (2009a) England and Wales. In: Hadfield, P (ed.), *Nightlife and crime*, pp. 19–50. Oxford: Oxford University Press.

Hadfield, P. and Measham, F. (2009b) Shaping the night: how licensing, social divisions and informal social controls mould the form and content of nightlife. *Crime Prevention and Community Safety* **11**, 219–34.

Haines, B. and Graham, K. (2005) Violence prevention in licensed premises. In: Stockwell, T., Gruenewald., P.J., Toumbourou, J.W. and Loxley, W. (eds), *Preventing harmful substance abuse*, pp. 163–76. Chichester: Wiley.

Halsey, A.H. (1986) *Change in British society.* Oxford: Oxford University Press.

Hamers, F.F., Batter, V., Downs, A.M., Alix, J., Cazein, F. and Brunet, J.B. (1997) The HIV epidemic associated with injecting drug use in Europe: geographic and time trends. *AIDS* **7**, 1365–74.

Hansen, W.B., Graham, J.W., Sobel, J.L., Shelton, D.R., Flay, B.R. and Johnson, C.A. (1987) The consistency of peer and parent influences on tobacco, alcohol and marijuana use among young adolescents. *Journal of Behavioral Medicine* **10**, 559–79.

Harms, E. (ed.) (1965) *Drug addiction in youth.* London: Pergamon.

Harris, C. (2005) Our city centres are abandoned to drunk, noisy louts. *The Times* 10 August, p. 2.

Harrison, BN. (1971) *Drink and the Victorians.* London: Faber and Faber.

Haw, S. and Higgins, K. (1998) A comparison of the prevalence of HIV infection and injecting risk behaviour in urban and rural samples in Scotland. *Addiction* **93**, 855–63.

Hawthorne, G. (2001) Drug education: myth and reality. *Drug and Alcohol Review* **20**, 111–19.

Hawthorne, G., Garrard, J. and Dunt, D. (1995) Does Life Education's drug education programme have a health benefit? *Addiction* **90**, 205–16.

Health Protection Agency, Health Protection Scotland, National Public Health Service for Wales, CDSC Northern Ireland and CRDHB (2006) *Shooting up: injections among injecting drug users in the United Kingdom 2005*, an update, October 2006. London: Health Protection Agency.

Heath, D. (ed.) (1995) *International handbook on alcohol and culture.* Westport, CT: Greenwood Press.

Heather, N., Rollnick, S. and Bell, A. (1993) Predictive validity of the Readiness to Change Questionnaire. *Addiction* **88**, 1667–77.

Heather, N. Wodak, A. and O'Hare, P. (eds) (2008) *Psychoactive drugs and harm reduction: From faith to science.* London: Whurr Publications.

Helzer, J.E., Robins, L.N., Taylor, J.R., Carey, K., Miller, R.H., Combs-Orme, T. and Farmer, A. (1985) The extent of long-term moderate drinking among alcoholics discharged from medical and psychiatric treatment facilities. *New England Journal of Medicine* **312**, 1678–82.

Hencke, D. and Sparrow, A. (2009) Gordon Brown rejects call to set minimum prices for alcohol. *The Guardian* 16 March, http://www.guardian.co.uk/politics/2009/mar/16/gordon-brown-alcohol-pricing

Herald (2007) Alcohol-related death rates 1998-2004. *Herald Newspaper*, Glasgow 23 February, p. 1.

Hersh, S.M. (2005) A powerbase of warlords. In: *Chain of command*, p. 155. Harmondsworth: Penguin.

Hess, L. (1995) Changing family patterns in Western Europe: Opportunities and risk factors for adolescent development. In: Rutter, M. and Smith, D. (eds), *Psychosocial disorders in young people: Time trends and their causes*, pp. 104–93. Chichester: Wiley.

Hibell, B. et al. (1997) *The 1995 ESPAD Report: Alcohol and other drug use amongst students in 26 European countries.* Stockholm: Swedish Council for Information on Alcohol and Other Drugs.

Hibell, B., Andersson, B., Balakireva, O., Bjarnasson, T., Kokkevi, A. and Morgan, M. (2000) *The 1999 ESPAD Report: Alcohol and other drug use among students in 30 European countries.* Stockholm: Swedish Council for Information on Alcohol and other Drugs.

Hibell, B., Andersson, B., Bjarnasson, T. Ahlström, S., Balakireva, O., Kokkevi, A. and Morgan, M. (2004) *The 2003 ESPAD Report: Alcohol and other drug use among students in 35 European countries.* Stockholm: Swedish Council for Information on Alcohol and other Drugs.

Hibell, B. Guttormsson, U., Ahlström, S., Balakireva, O., Bjarnasson, T., Kokkevi, A. and Kraus, L. (2009) *The 2007 ESPAD Report: Alcohol and other drug use among students in 35 European countries.* Stockholm: Swedish Council for Information on Alcohol and other Drugs.

Hickman, M., Higgins, V., Hope, V., Bellis, M., Tilling, K., Walker, A. and Henry, J. (2004) Injecting drug use in Brighton, Liverpool, and London: Best estimates of prevalence and coverage of public health indicators. *Journal of Epidemiology and Community Health* **5**, 766–71.

Hidimichi, Y., Nobuyuki, H. and Keitaro, M. (1999) Censoring and truncation in survival analysis. *Biotherapy* **13**, 811–16.

Higgins, K. and Kilpatrick, R. (2005) The impact of paramilitary violence against a heroin-user community in Northern Ireland: A qualitative analysis. *International Journal of Drug Policy* **16**, 334–42.

Higgins, K., Percy, A. and McCrystal, P. (2004) Secular trends in substance use: The conflict and young people in Northern Ireland. *Journal of Social Issues* **60**, 485–506.

Hillman, D.C.A. (2008) *The chemical muse: Drug use and the roots of Western civilisation.* New York: Thomas Dunne Books.

Hilton, T.F., Chandler, R.K. and Compton, W.M. (2008) Longitudinal research that can inform dynamic models for the treatment of addiction as a disease. *Evaluation Review* 32, 3–6.

Hindmarch, I. (1970) Patterns of drug use in a provincial university. *British Journal of Addiction* **64**, 395–403.

Hingson, R.W. and Kenkel, D. (2004) Social, health and economic consequences of underage drinking. In: *National Research Council and Institute of Medicine, Reducing underage drinking: A collective responsibility*, background papers, Committee on Developing a Strategy to Reduce and Prevent Underage Drinking, Division of Behavioural and Social Sciences and Education. Washington DC: The National Academies Press.

Hinscliff, G. (2008) Call for science to rule on risk of illegal drugs. *The Observer* 27 April, p. 4.

HM Government (1998) *Tackling drugs to build a better Britain: The Government's Ten-Year Strategy for Tackling Drugs.* London: Stationery Office.

HM Government (2008a) *Drugs: Protecting families and communities: The 2008 Drug Strategy.* London Home Office.

HM Government (2008b) *Drugs: Protecting families and communities: The 2008 Drug Strategy: Action Plan 2008-2011.* London: Home Office.

Hoare, J. (2009) *Drug misuse declared: Findings from the 2008/09 British Crime Survey: England and Wales.* London: Home Office, July, http://www.homeoffice.gov.uk/rds/pdfs09/hosb1209.pdf

Hoare, J. and Flatley, J. (2008) *Drug misuse declared: Findings from the 2007/08 British Crime Survey.* In Murphy, R. and Roe, S. (eds), *Drug misuse declared: Findings from the 2006/07 British Crime Survey*, Statistical Bulletin 18/7. London: Home Office.

Holford, P. and Cass, H. (2002) *Natural highs: Increase your energy, sharpen your mind, improve your mood, relax and beat stress with legal, natural and healthy mind-altering substances.* London: Piatkus.

Holland, J. (ed.) (2001) *Ecstasy: The complete guide.* Rochester, VT: Park Street Press.

Hollands, R. and Chatterton, P. (2001) *Changing our Toon: Youth, nightlife and urban change in Newcastle*. Newcastle: University of Newcastle.

Home Office (1971) *The Misuse of Drugs Act*. London: Home Office.

Home Office (1998) *Tackling drugs to build a better Britain*. London: Home Office.

Home Office (2002) *Updated drug strategy 2002*. London: Home Office.

Home Office (2003) *Drinking, crime and disorder*, Findings 185. London: Home Office.

Home Office (2004) *Arrests for notifiable offences and the operation of certain police powers under PACE*, Statistical Bulletin 18/04. London: Home Office.

Home Office Digest (2004) Cannabis is STILL illegal, p. 20. London: Home Office.

Home Office Online (2005a) Drug-assisted sexual assault, http://www.homeoffice.gov.uk/crime/sexualoffences/drug_assisted.html

Home Office Online (2005b) Cannabis reclassification, 28 January, http://www.homeoffice.gov.uk/publications/drugs/acmd1/cannabis-reclass-2005

Home Office Online (2008a) Crime reduction- helping reduce crime in your area. recent British crime reduction findings: drugs. http://www.crimereduction.homeoffice.gov.uk/drugsalcohol/drugsalcohol75.htm#Prevalence

Home Office Online (2008b) *Drug laws*, http://www.homeoffice.gov.uk/drugs/drugs-law/

Home Office Online (2008c) Drugs, protecting families and communities: The 2008 Drug Strategy. http://webarchive.nationalarchives.gov.uk/20100419081707/http://drugs.homeoffice.gov.uk/publication-search/drug-strategy/drug-strategy-2008ß

Homel, R., Hauritz, M., Wortley, R., Clark, J. and Carvolth, R. (1994a) *The impact of the surfers' paradise safety action project: Key findings of the evaluation*. Griffith University: Centre for Crime Policy and Public Safety.

Homel, R. and Clark, J. (1994b) The prediction and prevention of violence in pubs and clubs. *Crime Prevention Studies* **3**, 10–46.

Homel, R., Tomsen, S. and Thommeny, J. (1992) Public drinking and violence: not just an alcohol problem. *Journal of Drug Issues* **222**, 679–97.

Hood, L. (2009a) *Lessons learned from Nutt fallout*, 6 November, http://209.85.229.132/u/u we?q=cache:z808LI4PPlwJ:exquisitelife.researchresearch.com/exquisite_life/2009/11/lessons-learned-from-nutt-fallout.html

Hood, L. (2009b) Principles on the treatment of independent scientific advice provided to government, http://www.sciencecampaign.org.uk/documents/2009/CaSESTPrinciples.pdf

Hope, C. (2008) Use of extra strong "skunk" cannabis soars, *The Telegraph*, 6 February, http://www.telegraph.co.uk/news/uknews/1577798/Use-of-extra-strong-skunk-cannabis-soars.html

Hope, V.D., Hickman, M. and Tilling, K. (2005) Capturing crack cocaine use: estimating the prevalence of crack cocaine use in London using capture-recapture with covariates. *Addiction* **100**, 1701–8.

House of Commons Foreign Affairs Committee (2009) *Global security: Afghanistan and Pakistan*. London: House of Commons, 2 August, http://www.publications.parliament.uk/pa/cm200809/cmselect/cmfaff/302/302.pdf

House of Commons Public Administration Committee (2009) *Forty Seventh Report- Reducing alcohol harm: Health services in England for Alcohol Misuse*. London: House of Commons, 30 July, http://www.publications.parliament.uk/pa/cm200809/cmselect/cmpubacc/925/92502.htm

Hser, Y., Hoffman, V., Grella, C. and Anglin, D. (2001) A 33-year follow-up of narcotics addicts. *Archives of General Psychiatry* **58**, 503–8.

Huebner, A. and. Howell, L. (2003) Examining the relationship between adolescent sexual Risk-Taking and perceptions of monitoring, communication, and parenting styles. *Journal of Adolescent Health* **33**, 2, 71–8.

Hughes, K., Bellis, M. and Kilfoye-Carrington, M. (2001) *Alcohol, tobacco and drugs in the North West of England*. Liverpool: John Moores University.

Hughes, S., Bellis, M.A., Hughes, K., Tocque, K., Morleo, M., Hennessey, M. and Smallthwaite, L. (2008) *Risky drinking in North West school children and its consequences: A study of fifteen and sixteen year olds*. Liverpool: John Moores University.

Humphreys, K. (2004) *Circles of recovery: Self-help organisations for addictions*. Cambridge: Cambridge University Press.

Hutchinson, M., Jemmott, J., Sweet Jemmott, L., Braverman, P. and Fong, G. (2003) The role of mother–daughter sexual risk communication in reducing sexual risk behaviors among urban adolescent females: a prospective study. *Journal of Adolescent Health* **33**, 98–107.

Hutton, F. (2004) Up for it, mad for it? Women, drug use and participation in club scenes. *Health, Risk and Society* **6**, 223–37.

Hutton, F. (2006) *Risky pleasures? Club cultures and feminine identities*. Abingdon: Ashgate.

Hyman, S.E. (1996) Shaking out the cause of addiction. *Science* **273**, 611–12.

Inglis, B. (1975) *The forbidden game: A social history of drugs*. London: Coronet Books.

Institute of Medicine (1996) *Pathways of addiction: Opportunities in drug abuse research*. Washington DC: National Academy Press.

Interdepartmental Committee on Drug Addiction (1961) *Report of the report of the Interdepartmental Committee*. London: Ministry of Health, Scottish Home and Health Department.

Interdepartmental Committee on Drug Addiction (1965) *Second report: Report of the Interdepartmental Committee*. London: Ministry of Health, Scottish Home and Health Department.

International Drug Policy Consortium (2009) *Why is the outcome of the United Nations drug policy review so weak and inconclusive?*, IDPC briefing paper, 6 April, http://www.idpc. net/publications/why-is-outcome-of-un-drug-policy-review-so-weak-inconclusive

International Narcotics Control Board (2008a) *Report of the International Narcotics Control Board for 2007*. Lyons: International Narcotics Control Board, http://www.incb.org/ incb/annual-report-2007.html

International Narcotics Control Board (2008b) *Single Convention on Narcotic Drugs*, 1961, http://en.wikipedia.org/wiki/International_Opium_Convention

International Narcotics Control Board (2009a) *Single Convention on Narcotic Drugs*, 1961,http://www.incb.org/incb/convention_1961.html

International Narcotics Control Board (2009b) *Mandate and functions*, http://www.incb. org/incb/ru/mandate.html

Jackson, C., Henriksen, L. and Dickinson, D. (1999) Alcohol-specific socialization, parenting behaviours and alcohol use by children. *Journal of Studies on Alcohol* **60**, 362–7.

James, I.P. (1969) Delinquency and heroin addiction in Britain. *British Journal of Criminology* **9**, 108–24.

Järvinen, M. and Room, R (2007) Youth drinking cultures: European experiences. In: Järvinen, M. and Room, R. (eds), *Youth drinking cultures: European experiences*, pp. 1–16. Aldershot: Ashgate.

Jeffs, B. and Saunders, W. (1983) Minimising alcohol-related offences by enforcement of the existing legislation. *British Journal of Addiction* **78**, 67–78.

Jenkins, S. (2004) Labour has lost the plot on drugs. *Evening Standard* 15 January, p. 11.

Jenkins, S. (2007) Britain is stoned at home and sold out in Helmand. *The Guardian* 29 August, p. 29.

Jessor, R. and Jessor, S.L. (1977) *Problem behavior and psychosocial development: A longitudinal study of youth*. New York: Academic Press.

Jessor, R., Donovan, J.E. and Costa, F. (1991) *Beyond adolescence: Problem behavior and young adulthood*. New York: Cambridge University Press.

Johns, M.E., Brems, C. And Fisher, D.G. (1996) Self-reported levels of psychopathology of drug abusers not currently in treatment. *Journal of Psychopathology and Behavioral Assessment* **18**, 21–40.

Johnston, L., Bachman, J.G. and O'Malley, P.M. (1996) *Monitoring the future: national survey results on Drug Use 1995 Survey Data*. Bethesda, MD: National Institute on Drug Abuse.

Johnston, L., O'Malley, P.M. Bachman, J.G. and Schulenberg, J.E. (2004) *Monitoring the future: national survey results on Drug Use 1975-2003. Volume I: Secondary school students*. Bethesda, MD: National Institute on Drug Abuse. http://www.sundayherald.com/print47161

Johnston, L., O'Malley, P.M., Bachman, J.G. and Schulenberg, J.E. (2004) *Monitoring the future: national survey results on Drug Use 1975-2003, Volume II, College students and young adults*. Bethesda, MD: National Institute on Drug Abuse.

Jones, T. (1968) *Drugs and the police*. London: Butterworths.

Joseph Rowntree Foundation/DrugScope (2004) *Drug testing in the workplace: The report of the Independent Inquiry into Drug Testing at Work*. York: Joseph Rowntree Foundation/DrugScope.

Joseph Rowntree Foundation (2007) *New poverty and wealth maps of Britain reveal inequality to be at 40-year high*, 17 July, http://www.jrf.org.uk/pressroom/releases/170707.asp

Jotangia, D. and Thompson, J. (2009) Drug use. In: Fuller, E. (ed.), *Drug use, smoking and drinking among young people in England in 2008*, pp. 125–66. London: Health and Social Care Information Centre. http://www.ic.nhs.uk/webfiles/publications/sdd08full-report/SDD_England_2008_full_report.pdf

Kalb, M. (1975) The myth of alcoholism prevention. *Preventive Medicine* **4**, 404–16.

Kandel, D.B. (ed.) (1978) *Longitudinal research on drug use*. New York: Halstead.

Kimber, J., Copeland, L., Hickman, M., Macleod, J., McKenzie, J., De Angelis, D. and Robertson, J.R. (2010) Survival and cessation in injecting opiate users, a prospective observational study of outcomes and the effect of opiate substitute treatment. *British Medical Journal* (in press).

Kinder, B.N., Pape, N.E. and Walfish, S. (1980) Drug and alcohol education programs: a review of outcome studies. *International Journal of the Addictions* **15**, 1035–56.

King, L.A., Carpenties, C. and Griffiths. P. (2004) *An overview of cannabis potency in Europe.* Lisbon: European Monitoring Centre for Drugs and Drug Abuse.

Kirby, T. (2006) Laughing gas, the legal drug sweeping clubland that is making regulators frown. *The Independent* 14 January, http://www.independent.co.uk/life-style/health-and-wellbeing/health-news/laughing-gas-the-legal-drug-sweeping-clubland-that-is-making-regulators-frown-522919.html

Kohn, M. (1987) *Narcomania.* London: Faber and Faber.

Kohn, M. (1992) *Dope girls: The birth of the British drug underground.* London: Granta.

Kokkevi, A. (2007) Psychosocial correlates of substance use in adolescence: a cross-national study in six European countries. *Drug and Alcohol Dependence* **86**, 67–74.

Kokkevi, A. and Fotiou, A. (2009) The ESPAD psychosocial module. In: Hibell, B. Guttormsson, U., Ahlström, S., Balakireva, O., Bjarnasson, T., Kokkevi, A. and Kraus, L. (eds), *The 2007 ESPAD report: Alcohol and other drug use among students in 35 European countries*, pp. 172–83. Stockholm: Swedish Council for Information on Alcohol and other Drugs.

Kosviner, A., Mitcheson, M.C., Myers, K., Ogborne, A., Stimson, G.V. Zacune, J. and Edwards, G. (1968) Heroin use in a provincial town. *Lancet* **i**, 1189–92.

Kouimtsidis, C., Reynolds, M. and Tolland, E. (2003) Substance misuse among women attending family planning clinics in a rural area in Britain: prevalence and associated problems. *Drugs, Education, Prevention and Policy* **10**, 195–202.

Kraigher, D., Jagsch, R., Gombas, W. et al. (2005) Use of slow-release oral morphine for the treatment of opioid dependence. *European Addiction Research* **11**, 145–51.

Kreitman, N. (1986) Alcohol consumption and the preventive paradox. *British Journal of Addiction* **81**, 353–63.

Lader, M.H. and Higgit, A.C. (1986) Management of benzodiazepine dependence - update 1986. *Addiction* **81**, 7–10.

Lader, M., Tylee, A. and Donoghue, J. (2009) Withdrawing benzodiazepines in primary care. *CNS Drugs* **23**, 19–34.

Lahaut, V.M.H.C.J., Jansen, H.A., Van de Mheen, D. and Garretsen, H.F.L. (2002) Non-response bias in a sample survey on alcohol consumption. *Alcohol and Alcoholism* **37**, 256–60.

Langendam, M.W., Van Brussel, G., Coutinho, R.A. and Van Ameijden, E.J. (2000) Methadone maintenance and cessation of injecting drug use: Results from the Amsterdam Cohort Study. *Addiction* **94**, 591–600.

Latcham, R.W., Kreitman, N., Plant, M.A. and Crawford, A. (1984) Regional Variations in British Alcohol Morbidity Rates: A Myth Uncovered? I: Clinical Surveys. *British Medical Journal* **289**, 1341–3.

Laurie, P. (1967) *Drugs.* Harmondsworth: Penguin.

Ledoux, S., Miller, P., Choquet, M. and Plant, M.A. (2002) Family structure, parent-child relationships, and alcohol and other drug use among teenagers in France and the United Kingdom. *Alcohol & Alcoholism* **37**, 52–60.

Lefebure, M. (1974) *Samuel Taylor Coleridge: A bondage of opium.* New York: Stein and Day.

Left, S. (2003) Police bust UK's biggest ever cocaine ring. *The Guardian* 24 September, http://www.guardian.co.uk/uk/2003/sep/24/drugsandalcohol.colombia

Leith, S. (2009) We need a sensible debate about drugs- but that's impossible while ministers float above it all. *The Guardian G2* 12 February, p. 9.

Lemmens, P.H., Tan, E.S. and Knibbe, R.A. (1988) Bias due to non-response in a Dutch survey on alcohol consumption. *British Journal of Addiction* **83**, 1069–77.

Leung, S.F. and Yu, S. (2006) *Survey response bias and the determinants of substance use*, 11 July, https://editorialexpress.com/cgi-bin/conference/download.cgi?db_name=FEMES07&paper_id=341

Levine, H.G. (2003) Global drug prohibition: its uses and crises. *International Journal of Drug Policy* **14**, 145–53.

Levitt, R., Nason, E. and Hallsworth, M. (2006) *The evidence base for the classification of drugs*. Europe: RAND Corporation.

Lietava, J. (1992) Medicinal plants in a middle paleolithic grave Shanidar IV? *Journal of Ethnopharmacology* **35**, 263–6.

Lilywight, B. (1963) *London coffee houses*. London: Allen and Unwin.

Lindesmith, A.R. (1968) *Addiction and opiates*. Chicago: Aldine.

Lipsett, A. (2008) Schools may be judged on teenage pregnancy rates and drug problems. *The Guardian* 30 April, p. 1.

Liriano, S. and Ramsay, M. (2003) Prisoners' drug use before prison and the links with crime. In: Ramsay, M. (ed.), *Prisoners' drug use and treatment: Seven research studies*, Home Office Research Study 267. London: Home Office.

Lister, S., Hobbs, D., Hall, S. and Winslow, S. (2000) Violence in the night-time economy; bouncers: the reporting, recording and prosecution of assaults. *Policing and Society* **10**, 383–402.

Lloyd, T. (2010) Action needed to tackle social housing inequality. *Inside Housing*, 27 January, http://www.insidehousing.co.uk/story.aspx?storycode=6508265

London, M., O'Regan, T., Aust, P. and Stockford, A. (2006) Poppy tea drinking in East Anglia. *Addiction* **85**, 1345–7.

Lopez-Claros, A. and Zahidi, S. (2005) *Women's empowerment: Measuring the global gender gap*. Geneva: World Economic Forum.

Loretto, W. (1996) *Licit and illicit drug use in two cultures: A comparative study of adolescents in Scotland and Northern Ireland*, paper presented at 22nd Annual Alcohol Epidemiology Symposium. Edinburgh: Kettil Bruun Society, 6 June.

Lupton, R., Wilson, A., May, T., Warburton, H. and Turnbull, P.J. (2002) *A rock and a hard place: Drug markets in deprived neighbourhoods*, Home Office Research Study 240. London: Home Office.

MacAllister, W.B. (2000) *Drug Diplomacy in the Twentieth Century*. London: Routledge.

MacAndrew, C. and Edgerton, R.B. (1969) *Drunken Comportment: a Social Explanation*. Chicago: Aldine.

MacCoun, R. and Reuter, P. (2001) *Drug War Heresies: Learning from other Vices, Times and Places*. Cambridge: Cambridge University Press.

MacDonald, R. (2003) Crossing the Rubicon: youth transitions, poverty, drugs and social exclusion. *International Journal of Drug Policy* **13**, 27–9.

MacDonald, Z., Tinsley, L., Collingwood, J., Jamieson, P. and Pudney, S. (2005) *Measuring the Harm from Illegal Drugs Using the Drug Harm Index*, Home Office Online Reports 24/05. London: Home Office.

MacDonald, Z., Collingwood, J. and Gordon, L. (2006) Measuring the harm from illegal drugs using the harm index–an update, Home Office Online Reports 08/06. London: Home Office.

Macaulay, Lord (Thomas Babington) (1830) *Moore's Life of Lord Byron*. Whitefish, MT: Kessinger (republished in 2007).

MacGregor, S. (ed.) (1989) *Drugs in British Society*. London: Routledge.

Maden, A., Swinton, M. and Gunn, J. (1990) Women in prison and use of illicit drugs before arrest. *British Medical Journal* **301**, 1133.

Maden, A., Swinton, M. and Gunn, J. (1992) A survey of pre-arrest drug use in sentenced prisoners. *British Journal of Addiction* **87**, 27–33.

Maggs, J.L., Patrick, M.E. and Feinstein, L. (2008) Childhood and adolescent predictors of heavy drinking and alcohol use disorders in early adulthood: a longitudinal developmental analysis. *Addiction* **103**, 7–22.

Manning, P. (ed.) (2007) *Drugs and Popular Culture*. Uffculme, Devon: Willan Publishing.

Marks, H. (1997) *Mr Nice: An Autobiography*. London: Minerva.

Marmot, M. (2010) *Fair Society, Healthy Lives: Stategic Review of Health Inequalites in England Post 2010*. Geneva: World Health Organization, http://www.ucl.ac.uk/gheg/marmotreview/FairSocietyHealthyLives

Marsden, J. and Strang, J., with Lavoie, D., Abdulrahim, D., Hickman, M. and Scott, S. (2004a) Epidemiologically-based needs assessment: drug misuse. In: Stevens, A. and Rafferty, J. (eds), *Health Care Needs Assessment*. Oxford: Radcliffe.

Marsden, J., Strang, J., Scott, S. et. al. (2004b) Drug Misuse. In: Stevens, A,. Raferty, J., Mant, J. and Simpson, S. (eds), *Health Care Needs Assessment: The Epidemiologically Based Needs Assessment Review*. Oxford: Radcliffe.

Martin, P. (2008) *Sex, Drugs and Chocolate: The Science of Pleasure*. London: Fourth Estate.

Massing, M. (1998) *Fix: Solving the Nation's Drug Problem*. New York: Simon and Schuster.

Master, F. (2009) Drugs body pushes for ban on "herbal highs.' Reuters 12 August, http://uk.news.yahoo.com/22/20090812/tts-uk-herbal-ca02f96.html

Mathers, B.M., Degenhardt, L., Phillips, B., Wiessing, L., Hickman, M., Strathdee, S.A., Wodak, A., Panda, S., Tyndall., M, Toufik, A. and Mattick R.P. (2008) Global epidemiology of injecting drug use and HIV among people who inject drugs: a systematic review. *Lancet* **372**, 1733–45.

Matrix Knowledge Group (2007) *The Illicit Drug Trade in the United Kingdom*, Home Office Online Report 20/7. London: Home Office.

Matthews, P. (1999) *Cannabis Cultures: A Journey through Disputed Territory*. London: Bloomsbury.

Matthews, P. (2003) *Cannabis Culture*. London: Bloomsbury.

Mattick, R.P., Breen, C., Kimber, J. and Davoli, M. (2003) Methadone maintenance therapy versus no opioid replacement therapy for opioid dependence. *Cochrane Database of Systematic Reviews* **2**, CD002209.

Matza, D. (1964) *Delinquency and Drift*. New York: Wiley.

Matza, D. (1969) *Becoming Deviant*. Englewod Cliffs, NJ: Prentice Hall.

May, C. (2005) *The CARAT Drug Service in Prisons: Findings from the Research Database*, Findings 262. London: Home Office,

May, T., Warburton, H. and Turnbull, P. (2002) *Times They are a Changing: Policing of Cannabis*. York: Joseph Rowntree Foundation.

May, T., Duffy, M., Few, B. and Hough, M. (2005) *Understanding Drug selling in Communities: Insider or Outsider Trading?* York: Joseph Rowntree Foundation.

Mayo Clinic (2004) Marijuana: adverse effects. *Medical and Health Information for a Healthier Life* 30 January, http://www.mayoclinic.com

McAleney, J. and McMahon, J. (2006) Establishing rates of binge drinking in the UK: Anomalies in the data. *Alcohol & Alcoholism* **41**, 355–7.

McAulay, R. and Duffy, G. (2009) Junkie killed injecting anthrax. *The Scottish Sun* December 18, p. 1.

McBride, A.J. and Thomas, H. (1995) Psychosis is also common in users of "normal" cannabis. *British Medical Journal* **311**, 875.

McBride, N. (2005) The evidence base for school drug education interventions. In: Stockwell, T., Gruenewald, P.J., Toumbourou, J.W. and Loxley, W. (eds), *Preventing Harmful Substance Abuse*, pp. 101–12. Chichester: Wiley.

McCrystal, P. and Percy, A. (2009) A profile of adolescent cocaine use in Northern Ireland. *International Journal of Drug Policy* **20**, 357–64.

McDonald, M. (ed.) (1994) *Gender, Drink and Drugs: Cross Cultural Perspectives on Women*. Oxford/Providence: Berg.

Mc Ellrath, K. (2002) *Prevalence of Heroin Use in Northern Ireland*. Belfast: Drug and Alcohol Information & Research Unit.

Mc Ellrath, K. (2005) *Drug Use and Risk Behaviours among Injecting Drug Users*. Belfast: Drug and Alcohol Information & Research Unit.

Mc Ellrath, K. (2009) Northern Ireland. In: Hadfield, P (ed.), *Nightlife and Crime*, pp. 65–76. Oxford: Oxford University Press.

McElrath, M. (2004) Drug use and drug markets in the context of political conflict: The case of Northern Ireland. *Addiction Research & Theory* **12**, 577–90.

McGrath, M. (2008) Weed control. *Jane's Police Review* 13 June, 18–19

McGrath, Y., Sumnall, H., McVeigh, J. and Bellis, M. (2006) *Drug Use Prevention among Young People: A Review of Reviews*, evidence briefing update. London: National Institute for Health and Clinical Excellence.

McKeganey, N. (2005) *Random Drug Testing of Schoolchildren: A Shot in the Arm or a Shot in the Foot for Drug Prevention?* York: Joseph Rowntree Foundation.

McKenna, T. (1992) *Food of the Gods: The Secret for the Original Tree of Life: A Radical History of Plants, Drugs and Human Evolution*. New York: Bantam.

McLellan, A., Lewis, D., O'Brien, C. and Kleber, H. (2000) Drug dependence, a chronic medical illness: implications for treatment, insurance and outcomes evaluation. *Journal of the American Medical Association* **284**, 1689–95.

McMullan, S. and Ruddy, D. (2005) *Experience of Drug Misuse: Findings from the 2003/04 Northern Ireland Crime Survey*. Belfast: Statistics and Research Branch, Northern Ireland Office.

McSweeney, T., Turnbull, P.J. and Hough, M. (2008) *Tackling Drug Markets and Distribution Networks in the UK*. London: UK Drug Policy Commission.

Measham, F. (2002) Doing drugs, doing gender: conceptualising the gendering of drugs cultures. *Contemporary Drug Problems* **29**(2), 335–73.

Measham, F. (2004) The decline of ecstasy, the rise of 'binge' drinking and the persistence of pleasure. *Probation Journal* **5**, 309–26.

Measham, F., Newcombe, R. and Parker, H. (1994) The normalization of recreational drug use amongst young people in North-West England. *The British Journal of Sociology* **45**, 287–312.

Meier, P., Brennan, A., Purshouse, R., Taylor, K., Rafia, R., Booth, A., O'Reilly, D., Stockwell, T., Sutton, A., Wilkinson, A. and Wong, R. (2008) *Independent Review of the Effects of Alcohol Pricing and Promotion: Part B: Modelling the Potential Impact of Pricing and Promotion Policies for Alcohol in England: Results from the Sheffield Alcohol Policy Model Version 2008 (1-1)*, http://www.dh.gov.uk/en/Publichealth/ Healthimprovement/Alcoholmisuse/DH_4001740

Meier, P., Purshouse, R., Meng, Y., Rafia, R. and Brennan, A. (2009) *Model Based Appraisal of Alcohol Minimum Pricing and off Licensed Trade Discount Bans in Scotland: A Scottish Adaptation of the Sheffield Alcohol Policy Model*. Sheffield: University of Sheffield.

Merline, A., Jager, J. and Schulenberg, J.E. (2008) Adolescent risk factors for adult alcohol use and abuse: stability and change of predictive value across early and middle adulthood. *Addiction* **103**, 84–99.

Midford, R. and McBride, N. (2004) Alcohol education in schools. In: Heather, N. and Stockwell, T. (eds), *The Essential Handbook of Treatment and Prevention of Alcohol Problems*, pp. 299–319. John Wiley: West Sussex.

Milgram, G. (1976) A historical review of alcohol education research and comments. *Journal of Alcohol & Drug Education* **21**, 1–16.

Milgram, G. (1987) Alcohol and drug education programs. *Journal of Drug Education* **17**, 43–57.

Millar, T., Gemmell, I., Hay, G., Heller, R.F. and Donmall, M. (2006) How well do trends in incidence of heroin use reflect hypothesised trends in prevalence of problem drug use in the North West of England? *Addiction Research and Theory* **14**, 537–49.

Miller, P. (1997) Family structure, personality, drinking, smoking and illicit drug use: a study of UK teenagers. *Drug and Alcohol Dependence* **45**, 121–9.

Miller, P. and Plant, M.A. (1996) Drinking, smoking and illicit drug use amongst 15-16 year olds: a UK study. *British Medical Journal* **313**, 394–7.

Miller, P. and Plant, M.A. (1999) Truancy, perceived school performance, family structure, lifestyle, alcohol, cigarettes and illicit drugs: a study of UK teenagers. *Alcohol & Alcoholism* **34**, 886–93.

Miller, P. and Plant, M.A. (1999) Use and perceived ease of obtaining illicit drugs amongst teenagers in urban, suburban and rural schools: a UK study. *Journal of Substance Use* **4**, 24–8.

Miller, P. and Plant, M.A. (2001a) Drinking and smoking among 15 and 16 year olds in the United Kingdom: a re-examination. *Journal of Substance Use* **5**, 285–9.

Miller, P. and Plant, M.A. (2001b) *Drinking, Smoking and Illicit Drug Use amongst 15 and 16 year old School Students in Northern Ireland*, report for Department of Health, Social Services and Public Safety, Belfast. Edinburgh: Alcohol & Health Research Centre.

Miller, P. and Plant, M.A. (2002) Heavy cannabis use among UK teenagers: an exploration. *Drug and Alcohol Dependence* **65**, 235–42.

Miller, P. and Plant, M.A. (2003a) Teenage beverage preferences: Risk and responses. *Health, Risk and Society* **5**, 3–10.

Miller, P. and Plant, M.A. (2003b) The family, peer influences and substance use among UK teenagers. *Journal of Substance Use* **8**, 19–26.

Miller, P. and Plant, M.A. (2004) *The Reclassification of Cannabis: Knowledge and Opinions of UK Teenagers*, unpublished report for the Joseph Rowntree Foundation. Bristol: Alcohol & Health Research Trust.

Miller, P. and Plant, M.A. (2010) Parental guidance about drinking: Relationship with teenage psychoactive substance use. *Journal of Adolescence* **33**, 55–68.

Miller, P., Plant, M.A., Choquet, M. and Ledoux, S. (2002) Cigarettes, alcohol, drugs and self-esteem: A comparison of 15-16 year olds from France and the United Kingdom. *Journal of Substance Use* **7**, 71–7.

Mills, J.H. (2003) *Cannabis Britannica: Empire, Trade and Prohibition*. Oxford: Oxford University Press.

Mohler-Kuo, M., Dowdall, G., Koss, M. and Weschler, H. (2004) Correlates of rape while intoxicated in a sample of college women. *Journal of Studies on Alcohol* **65**, 37–45.

Mohr A.F. (2000) Adolescent substance-abuse: Vulnerability and protective factors from a developmental perspective. *Dissertation Abstracts International Section A: Humanities & Social Sciences* **60**(7-A), 2373.

Møller, L., Heino Stöver, H., Jürgens, R., Gatherer, A. and Nikogosian, H. (eds) (2007) *Health in Prisons A WHO Guide to the Essentials in Prison Health*. Geneva: World Health Organization.

Morgan, C.J.A., Muetzelfeldt, L., Muetzelfeldt, M., Nutt, D.F. and Curran, H.V. (2010) Harms associated with psychoactive substances: findings of the UK National Drug Survey. *Journal of Psychopharmacology* **24**, 147–53.

MORI (1979) Survey of drug use carried out for *Now! Magazine*. London: MORI.

Morris, N. (2007) Former prisons inspector backs call to legalise drugs. *The Independent* 16 October, http://www.independent.co.uk/news/uk/politics/former-prisons-inspector-backs-call-to-legalise-drugs-396961.html

Morris, S., Humphreys, D. and Reynolds, D. (2006) Myth, marula, and elephant: An assessment of voluntary ethanol intoxication of the African Elephant (*Loxodonta africana*) following feeding on the fruit of the marula tree (*Sclerocarya birrea*). *Physiological and Biochemical Zoology* **79**, 363–9.

Mott, J. (1985) Self-reported cannabis use in Great Britain in 1981. *British Journal of Addiction* **80**, 30–43.

Mott, J. and Rathod, N.H. (1976) Heroin misuse and delinquency in a new town. *British Journal of Psychiatry* **128**, 428–35.

Mounts, N.S. (2000) Parental management of adolescent peer relationships: what are its effects on friend selection? In: Kerns, K., Contreras, J.M. and Neal-Barnett, A.M. (eds), *Family and Peers: Linking Two Social Worlds*, pp. 167–93. Westport: Praeger.

Murphy, R. and Roe, S. (2007) *Drug Misuse Declared: Findings from the 2006/07 British Crime Survey*, Statistical Bulletin 18/7. London: Home Office.

Murray, R. (2007) Teenage schizophrenia is the issue, not legality. *Independent on Sunday* 18 March, http://www.independent.co.uk/opinion/commentators/robin-murray-teenage-schizophrenia-is-the-issue-not-legality-440670.html

Musto, D. (1987) *The American Disease: Origins of Narcotic Control*. New York: Oxford University Press.

Musto, D. (1997) Alcohol control in historical perspective. In: Plant, M.A., Single, E. and Stockwell, T. (eds), *Alcohol: Minimising the Harm: What Works?*, pp. 10–25 London: Free Association Books.

Nadelmann, E. (2009) International Narcotics Control Board reaffirms its shameful commitment to politics over science. *Huffington Post* 19 February, http://www.huffingtonpost.com/ethan-nadelmann/international-narcotics-c_b_168352.html

Nadelmann, E., McNeely, J. and Drucker, E. (1997) Harm reduction drug control strategies: a global perspective. In: Lowinson, J., Ruiz, P. and Millman, R. (eds), *Substance Abuse: a Comprehensive Textbook*, pp. 22–39. Baltimore, MD: Williams and Wilkins.

Natarajan, M. and Hough, M. (eds.) (2004) *Illegal Drug Markets*. Uffculme, Devon: Willan Publishing.

National Assembly for Wales (2000) *Tackling Substance Misuse in Wales: a Partnership Approach*. Cardiff, National Assembly for Wales.

National Centre for Social Research (2010) 2007 *British Social Attitudes Survey*. London: National Centre for Social Research.

National Centre for Social Research/National Foundation for Educational Research (2005) *Smoking, Drinking and Drug Use among Young People in England in 2004*. London: National Centre for Social Research/National Foundation for Educational Research.

National Equality Panel (2010) *An anatomy of the economic inequality in the UK*. London. National Inequality Panel.

National Institute for Health and Clinical Excellence (NICE) (2007a) *Drug Misuse: Opiate Detoxification*, NICE Clinical Guideline 52. London: National Institute for Health and Clinical Excellence.

National Institute for Health and Clinical Excellence (NICE) (2007b) *Drug Misuse: Psychosocial Interventions*, NICE Clinical Guideline 51. London: National Institute for Health and Clinical Excellence.

National Institute for Health and Clinical Excellence (NICE) (2007c) *Naltrexone for the Management of Opioid Dependence*, NICE Technology Appraisal Guidance 115. London: National Institute for Health and Clinical Excellence.

National Institute for Health and Clinical Excellence (NICE) (2007d) *Methadone and Buprenorphine for the Management of Opioid Dependence*, NICE Technology Appraisal 114. London: National Institute for Health and Clinical Excellence.

National Institute on Drug Abuse (2003) *Preventing Drug Use among Children and Adolescents*, 2nd edn. Bethesda, MD: National Institute on Drug Abuse.

National Treatment Agency for Substance Misuse (NTA) (2002) *Models of Care for Treatment of Adult Drug Misusers*. London: National Treatment Agency for Substance Misuse.

Neale, J. (2002) *Drug Users in Society*. London: Palgrave.

Newburn, T. and Shiner, M. (2001) *Teenage Kicks? Young People and Alcohol: A Review of the Literature*. York: Joseph Rowntree Foundation.

Newbury-Birch, D., Walshaw, D. and Kamali, F. (2001) Drink and drugs: from medical students to doctors. *Drug and Alcohol Dependence* **64**, 265–70.

New Scientist (2006) Timeline: Drugs and Alcohol, 4 September, http://www.newscientist.com/channel/being-human/drugs-alcohol/dn9924-timeline.dr

NHS Confederation (2010) *Too Much of the Hard Stuff: What Alcohol Costs the NHS*. London: Royal College of Physicians.

Nicholls, J. (2009) *The Politics of Alcohol*. Manchester: Manchester University Press.

NOP Market Research Ltd. (1982) Survey of drug use in the 15-21 age group undertaken for the Daily Mail. London: NOP.

Northern Ireland Office (1999) *Drug Strategy for Northern Ireland*. Belfast, Northern Ireland Office.

Norton, S. (2005) The origins of pharmacology in the 16th Century. *Molecular Interventions* **5**, 144–9.

Number 10 (2010) *Back-Prof-Nutt - Epetition Response*, 2 February, http://www.number10.gov.uk/Page22548

Nutt, D.J. (1986) Benzodiazepine dependence in the clinic: reason for anxiety? *Trends in Pharmacological Sciences* 7, 457–60.

Nutt, D.J. (2009a) Equasy — An overlooked addiction with implications for the current debate on drug harms. *Journal of Psychopharmacology* **23**, 3–5.

Nutt, D. (2009b) *Estimating Drug Harms: A Risky Business?*, Briefing 10. London: Centre for Crime and Justice Studies.

Nutt, D. (2010) Reply to "Nutt damage". *Lancet* **375**, 724.

Nutt, D.J., King, L.A., Saulsbury, W. and Blakemore, C. (2007) Development of a rational scale to assess the harm of drugs of potential misuse. *The Lancet* **369**, 1047–53.

O'Brien, C. and Scott, J. (2007) The role of the family. In: Coleman, J. and Hagell, A. (eds), *Adolescence, Risk and Resilience: Against the Odds*, pp. 17–39. Chichester: Wiley.

O'Brien, C.P., Childress, A.R., Ehrman, R. and Robbins, S.J. (1998) Conditioning factors in drug abuse: can they explain compulsion? *Journal of Psychopharmacology* **12**, 15–22.

O'Farrell, T.J. and Fals-Stewart, W. (2006) *Behavioral Couples Therapy for Alcoholism and Drug Abuse*, New York: Guildford.

Office for National Statistics (2006) *Health Statistics Quarterly* 23 February, (Spring 2006), http://64.233.183.104/u/uwe?q=cache:chAOA3Tg-gUJ:www.gnn.gov.uk/imagelibrary/downloadMedia.asp%3FMediaDetailsID%3D148388+drugs,+occupation,+England&hl=en&ct=clnk&cd=3&ie=UTF-8

Office for National Statistics (2007) Bar staff and publicans have the highest proportions of alcohol-related deaths. *Health Statistics Quarterly* 23 August, (Autumn 2007), http://64.233.183.104/u/uwe?q=cache:DmiTbh_PSzQJ:www.statistics.gov.uk/pdfdir/hsq0807.pdf+alcohol,+occupation,+ONS&hl=en&ct=clnk&cd=1&ie=UTF-8

Office for National Statistics (2008a) *Drug Poisoning: Drug Deaths Lowest Since 1995*, http://www.statistics.gov.uk/cci/nugget.asp?id=806

Office for National Statistics (2008b) *General Household Survey 2006*, http://www.statistics.gov.uk/downloads/theme_compendia/GHS06/AppendixG2006.pdf,

O'Hare, P., Newcombe, R., Matthews, A., Buning, E.C. and Drucker, E. (eds) (1992) *The Reduction of Drug-related Harm*. London: Tavistock/Routledge.

Oliver, I. (2006) *Drug Affliction: All You Need to Know about Drugs*. Aberdeen: Robert Gordon University.

Oliver, P. and Keen, J. (2003) Concomitant drugs of misuse and drug using behaviours associated with fatal opiate-related poisonings in Sheffield, UK, 1997–2000. *Addiction* **98**, 191–7.

Oobject (2008) Drug Smuggling Submarines, http://www.oobject.com/category/drug-smuggling-submarines/

Orford, J., Natera, G., Copoello, A., Atkinson, C., Mora, J., Velleman, R., Crundall, I., Tiburcio, M., Templeton, L. and Walley, G. (2005) *Coping with Alcohol and Drug Problems.* London: Routledge.

Organisation for Economic Co-operation and Development (2009) *Doing Better for Children*, http://www.oecd.org/document/12/0,3343,en_2649_34819_43545036_1_1_1_37419,00.html

Owen, R.T. and Tyrer, P. (1983) Benzodiazepine dependence: a review of the evidence. *Drugs* **25**, 385–98.

Parker, H. (2005) Normalization as a barometer: Recreational drug use and the consumption of leisure by younger Britons. *Addiction Research and Theory* **13**, 205–15.

Parker, H. and Williams, L. (2001) Intoxicated weekends: Young adults' work hard, play hard lifestyles, public health and Public Disorder. *Drugs: Education, Prevention and Policy* **40**, 345–68.

Parker, H. and Egginton, R. (2002) Adolescent recreational alcohol and drug careers gone wrong: Developing a strategy for reducing risks and harms. *International Journal of Drug Policy* **13**, 4119–4423.

Parker, H., Newcombe, R. and Bakx, K. (1987) The new heroin users; prevalence and characteristics in Wirrell, Merseyside. *British Journal of Addiction* **82**, 147–57.

Parker, H., Bakx, K. and Newcombe, R. (1988) *Living With Heroin.* Milton Keynes: Open University Press.

Parker, H., Aldridge, J. and Measham, F. (1998) *Illegal Leisure: The Normalisation of Adolescent Drug Use.* London: Routledge.

Parker, H., Aldridge, J. and Eggington, R. (2001) *UK Drugs Unlimited: New Research and Policy Lessons on Illicit Drug Use.* Basingstoke: Palgrave.

Parrott, A., Milani, R.M., Parmar, R. and Turner, J.J.D. (2001) Recreational ecstasy/MDMA and other drug users from the UK and Italy: psychiatric symptoms and psychobiological problems. *Psychopharmacology* **159**, 77–82.

Parrott, A., Morinan, A., Moss, M. and Scholey, A. (2005) *Understanding Drugs and Behaviour.* London: Wiley.

Patience, M. (2009) Drug abuse hampers Afghan police. *BBC News Online* 18 February, http://news.bbc.co.uk/1/hi/world/south_asia/7895612.stm

Patton, G., Coffey, C., Carlin, J.B., Degenhardt, L., Lynskey, M. and Hall, W. (2002) Cannabis use and mental health in young people: cohort study. *British Medical Journal* **23**, 1195–8.

Patton, G.C., Coffey, C., Sawyer, S.M., Viner, R.M., Haller, D.M., Bose, K., Vos, T., Ferguson, J. and Mathers, C.D. (2009) Global patterns of mortality in young people: a systematic analysis of population health data. *Lancet* **374**, 881–92.

Payne, J. (2007) Women drug users in North Cumbria: what influences initiation into heroin in this non-urban setting. *Sociology of Health and Illness* **29**, 633–55.

Peck, S.C., Vida, M. and Eccles, J.S. (2008) Adolescent pathways to adult drinking: sport activity involvement is not necessarily risky or protective. *Addiction* **103**, 69–83.

Perle, R.F. (2001) *Taliban and the Drug Trade*, CRS Report for Congress, Congressional Research Service, the Library of Congress, 5 October, http://www.fpc.state.gov/documents/organization/6210.pdf

Peto, R., Lopez, A.D., Boreham, J., Thun, M. and Heath, C.J. (2004) *Mortality from Smoking in Developed Countries 1950–2000: Indirect Estimates from National Vital Statistics.* Oxford: MRC/Cancer Research UK/BHF Clinical Trial Service Unit.

Petry, N.M. (2000) Effects of income on polysubstance abuse: a comparison of alcohol, cocaine, and heroin abusers. *Addiction* **95**, 706–17.

Petry, N.M. (2001) A behavioral analysis of polysubstance abuse in alcoholics: asymmetrical substitution of alcohol and cocaine. *Drug and Alcohol Dependence* **62**, 31–9.

Petursson, H. and Lader, M.H. (1981) Benzodiazepine dependence. *British Journal of Addiction* **76**, 133–45.

Petzel, T.P., Johnson, J.E. and McKillip, A. (1973) Response bias in drug surveys. *Journal of Consulting and Clinical Psychology* **40**, 437–9.

Phillipson, R.V. (ed.) (1970) *Modern Trends in Drug Dependence and Alcoholism.* London: Butterworths.

Phipps R. (2005) *Addiction within a Northern Ireland Context*, paper presented at International Addictions Conference Exploring Research, Policy and Practice, Jordanstown Campus, University of Ulster, 7 September.

Pickens, K. (1985) Drug education: The effects of giving information. *Journal of Alcohol & Drug Education* **30**, 32–44.

Piontek, D., Kraus, L. and Klempova, D. (2008a) Short scales to assess cannabis-related problems: a review of psychometric properties. *Substance Abuse Treatment, Prevention and Policy* **3**, 25.

Piontek, D., Kraus, L. and Pabst, A. (2008b) The ESPAD cannabis module: cannabis-related problems amongst adolescents in 17 ESPAD countries. In: Hibell, B. Guttormsson, U., Ahlström, S., Balakireva, O., Bjarnasson, T., Kokkevi, A. and Kraus, L. (eds), *The 2007 ESPAD Report: Alcohol and other drug Use among Students in 35 European Countries*, pp. 164–70. Stockholm: Swedish Council for Information on Alcohol and other Drugs.

Pine, A. (2008) *Working Hard, Drinking Hard, On Violence and Survival in Honduras.* Berkley, University of California Press.

Pitkänen, T., Lyyra, A.-L. and Pulkkinen, L. (2005) Age of onset of drinking and the use of alcohol in adulthood: a follow-up study from age 8–42 for females and males. *Addiction* **100**, 652–61.

Pitkänen, T., Kokka, K., Lyyra, A.-L. and Pulkkinen, L. (2008) A developmental approach to alcohol drinking behaviour in adulthood: a follow-up study from age 8 to age 42. *Addiction* **103**, 48–68.

Plant, M.A. (1975) *Drugtakers in an English Town.* London: Tavistock.

Plant, M.A. (1979) *Drinking Careers: Occupations, Drinking Habits and Drinking Problems.* London: Tavistock.

Plant, M.A. (1981) *Drugs in Perspective*, Teach Yourself Series. London: Hodder and Stoughton.

Plant, M.A. (1989a) The Epidemiology of Illicit Drug Use and Misuse in Britain. In: MacGregor, S. (ed.), *Drugs in British Society*, pp. 52–64. London: Routledge.

Plant, M.A. (1989b) Some issues in the epidemiology of alcohol use and misuse. In: Plant, M.A. (ed.), *Alcohol-Related Problems in High Risk Groups*, pp. 1–31. Copenhagen: World Health Organization.

Plant, M.A. (ed.) (1990) *AIDS, Drugs and Prostitution*. London: Tavistock/Routledge.

Plant, M.A. (1999) ESPAD: The European School Survey Project on Alcohol & Other Drugs, *Alcohol Update*, Issue 40, 2–3. Glasgow: Scottish Council on Alcohol.

Plant, M.A. (2000) Young people and alcohol use. In: Aggleton, P., Hurry, J. and Warwick, I. (eds), *Young People and Mental Health*, pp. 13–28. London: Wiley.

Plant, M.A. (2001) Learning by experiment. In: Grant, M. (ed.), *Learning about Drinking*, International Center for Alcohol Policies Series on Alcohol in Society, pp. 129–46. Philadelphia: Brunner/Mazel.

Plant, M.A. (2004a) The Alcohol Harm Reduction Strategy for England: Overdue final report omits much that was useful in interim report. *The British Medical Journal* **328**, 905–6

Plant, M.A. and Reeves, C.E. (1973a) Social characteristics of drugtakers in two English urban areas. *Drugs and Society* **2**(11), 14–18.

Plant, M.A. and Reeves, C.E. (1973b) The group dynamics of becoming a drugtaker. *Interpersonal Development* **4**, 99–106.

Plant, M.A. and Ritson, E.B. (1976) The Scottish drug scene. *Health Bulletin* **34**(1), 12–15.

Plant, M.A. and Plant, M.L. (1992) *Risk Takers: Alcohol, Drugs, Sex and Youth*. London: Tavistock.

Plant, M.A. and Miller, P. (2000) Drug use has declined among teenagers in the UK. *British Medical Journal* **320**, 1536–7.

Plant, M.A. and Miller, P. (2001a) UK youth are heaviest drug users in Europe-again. *Substance Misuse Bulletin* **14**, 2–3.

Plant, M.A. and Miller, P. (2001b) *The 1999 European School Survey Project on Alcohol & other Drugs*, Alcohol Insight no 11. London: Alcohol Education & Research Council.

Plant, M.A. and Plant, M.L. (2001c) Young people and alcohol. *Nursing Times Research* **6**, 887–96.

Plant, M.A. and Plant, M.L. (2006) *Binge Britain: Alcohol and the National Response*. Oxford: Oxford University Press.

Plant, M.A. and Miller, P. (2007) Being 'taught to drink:' UK teenagers' experience. In: Järvinen, M. and Room, R. (eds), *Youth Drinking Cultures*, pp. 131–44. Aldershot: Ashgate.

Plant, M.A., Peck, D. and Samuel, E. (1985) *Alcohol, Drugs and School-Leavers*. London: Tavistock.

Plant, M.A. Goos, C., Keup, W. and Österberg, E. (eds.) (1990) *Alcohol and Drugs: Research and Policy*. Edinburgh: Edinburgh University Press.

Plant, M.A., Ritson, B. and Robertson, J.R. (eds) (1992) *Alcohol and Drugs: The Scottish Experience*. Edinburgh: Edinburgh University Press.

Plant, M.A., Single, E. and Stockwell, T. (eds) (1997) *Alcohol: Minimising the Harm: What Works?* London: Free Association Books.

Plant, M.A., Plant, M.L., Thornton, C. and Garretsen, H. (2000) Consequences: Patterns and trends. In: Plant, M.A. and Cameron, D. (eds), *The Alcohol Report*, pp. 130–9. London: Free Association Books.

Plant, M.A., Wilkinson, S. and Plant, M.L. (2002) *Mental Health Needs in Four Penal Institutions*. Bristol: University of the West of England.

Plant, M.A., Miller, P. and Plant, M.L. (2005) Trends in drinking, smoking and illicit drug use among 15 and 16 year olds in the United Kingdom (1995-2003). *Journal of Substance Use* **10**, 331–9.

Plant, M.L. (1985) *Women, Drinking and Pregnancy*. London: Tavistock.

Plant, M.L. (1997) *Women and Alcohol: Contemporary and Historical Perspectives*. London: Free Association Books.

Plant, M.L. and Plant, M.A. (2001) International researchers work together. *Substance Misuse Bulletin* **14**, 6–7.

Plant, M.L. and Plant, M.A. (eds) (2008) *Addiction: Major Themes in Health and Welfare* (four volumes). London: Routledge.

Plant, M.L., Plant, M.A. and Foster, J. (1991) Alcohol, tobacco and illicit drug use amongst nurses: A Scottish study, *Drug and Alcohol Dependence* **28**, 195–202.

Plant, M.L., Plant, M.A. and Mason, W. (2002a) Drinking, smoking and illicit drug use amongst British adults: gender differences explored. *Journal of Substance Use* **7**, 24-33.

Plant, M.L., Miller, P. and Plant, M.A. (2004) Childhood and adult sexual abuse: relationships with alcohol and other drug use. *Child Abuse Review* **13**, 200–14.

Plant, M.L. Miller, P. and Plant, M.A. (2005a) The relationship between alcohol consumption and problem behaviours: gender differences among British adults. *Journal of Substance Use* **10**, 22–30.

Plant, M.L., Plant, M.A. and Miller, P. (2005b) Childhood and adult sexual abuse: Relationships with 'addictive' or 'problem behaviours' and health. *Journal of Addictive Diseases* **24**, 25–38.

Plant, S. (1999) *Writing on Drugs*. London: Faber and Faber.

Police Foundation (2000) *Drugs and the Law: Report of the Independent Inquiry into the Misuse of Drugs Act 1971*. London: Police Foundation.

Pompidou Group (Council of Europe) (2006) *Young People and Drugs: Care and Treatment*. Warsaw: National Bureau for Drug Prevention, Poland.

Potter, D.J., Clark, P. and Brown, M.B. (2008) Cannabis in England in 2005: Implications for psychoactivity and pharmacology. *Journal of Forensic Sciences* **53**, 90–4.

Poulin, C. and Nicholson, J. (2005) Should harm minimization as an approval to adolescent substance use be embraced by junior and senior high schools?" *International Journal of Drug Policy* **16**, 403–14.

Powell, J., Steriou, A., Plant, M.A. and Miller, P. (2006) Drinking, smoking and illicit drug use among 15 and 16 year olds in the Isle of Man. *Journal of Substance Use* **11**, 1–10.

President of the Council (1998) *Tackling Drugs to Build a Better Britain: The Government's Ten-Year Strategy for Tackling Drugs Misuse*. London: The Stationary Office.

Pudney, S.E., Badillo, C., Bryan, M., Burton, J., Conti, G. and Iacovou, M. (2006) Estimating the size of the UK illicit drugs market. In: *Measuring Different Aspects of Problem Drug Use: Methodological Developments*, Home Office Online Report 16/06, pp. 46–120. London: Home Office.

Rabin, R. and de Charro, F. (2001) EQ-5D: a measure of health status from the EuroQol Group. *Annals of Medicine* **33**, 337–43.

Ramsay, M., Baker, P., Goulden, C., Sharp, C. and Sondhi, A. (2001) *Drug Misuse Declared in 2000: Results from the British Crime Survey*, Research Study 197. London: Home Office.

RAND (2003) *Study Links Early Alcohol Use and Behavior Problems in Young Adulthood* (press release), 5 May, http://www.jointogether.org/news/research/pressreleases/2003/study-links-early-alcohol-use.html

Rathod, N.H., Addenbrooke, W.M. and Rosenbach, A.F. (2005) Heroin dependence in an English town: 33-year follow-up. *British Journal of Psychiatry* **187**, 421–5.

Reed, L. (1964) Lyrics from Heroin. *The Velvet Underground and Nico* (1967), Verve Records (now Universal Music Group, New York).

Reuter, P and Stevens, A. (2007) *An Analysis of UK Drug Policy: A Monograph Prepared for the UK Drug Policy Commission*. London: UK Drug Policy Commission.

Rhodes, T. (1990) The politics of anti-drug campaigns. *Druglink* **5**, 16–19.

Richardson, A. and Budd, T. (2003) *Alcohol, Crime and Disorder: a Study of Young Adults*, Home Office Research Study Number 263. London: Home Office.

Riley, S. and Hayward, E. (2004) Patterns, trends and meanings of drug use by dance drug users in Edinburgh, Scotland. *Drugs: Education, Prevention and Policy* **11**, 243–62.

Ritson, E.B. (1971) Drug use in the provinces. *Drugs and Society* **2**, 19–24.

Robbins, C., Enev, T., O'Connell, D., Gealt, R.E. and Martin, S. (2008) *Gender, Parental Control and Adolescent Drug Use: A Reexamination of Power-Control Theory*, paper presented at Annual Meeting of the American Society of Criminology, Toronto.

Roberts, C., Moore, L., Blakey, V., Playle, R. and Tudor-Smith, C. (1995) Drug use among 15-16 year olds in Wales, 1990-1994. *Drugs: Education, Prevention and Policy* **2**, 305–16.

Roberts, K. (1983) *Youth and Leisure*. London: Allen and Unwin.

Robertson, J.R. (1986) *Heroin, AIDS and Society*. London: Hodder and Stoughton.

Robertson, J.R. and Richardson, A. (2007) Heroin injecting and the introduction of HIV/AIDS into a Scottish city. *Journal of the Royal Society of Medicine* **100**, 491–4.

Robertson, J.R., Bucknall, A.B., Welsby, P.D., Roberts, J.J., Inglis, J.M., Peutherer, J.F. and Brettle, R.P. (1986) Epidemic of AIDS related virus (HTLV-III/LAV) infection among intravenous drug abusers. *British Medical Journal (Clinical Research Ed)* **292**, 527–9.

Robertson, J.R., Macleod, J., Hickman, M., Copeland, L., McKenzie, J. and Kimber, J. (2010) The Edinburgh Addiction Cohort: Recruitment and follow-up of a primary care based sample of injection drug users and non drug-injecting controls. *BMC Medical Research Methodology* (under preparation).

Robins, L.N. (1966) *Deviant Children Grow Up*. Baltimore, MD: Williams and Wilkins.

Robins, L.N. (1973) *A Follow-up of Vietnam Drug Users*. Special Action Office Monograph, Series A, No. 1. Washington DC: Executive Office of the President.

Robins, L.N. (1974) *The Vietnam Drug User Returns*. Special Action Office Monograph, Series A, No. 2. Washington DC: U.S. Government Printing Office.

Robins, L.N. (1975) Drug treatment after return in Vietnam veterans. *Highlights of the 20th Annual Conference*, Veterans Administration Studies in Mental Health and Behavioral Sciences. Perry Point, MD: Central NP Research Laboratory.

Robins, L.N., Davis, D.H. and Nurco, D.N. (1974) How permanent was Vietnam drug addiction? *American Journal of Public Health* **64** (Suppl), 38–43.

Robins, L.N., Helzer, J.E. and Davis, D.H. (1975) Narcotic use in Southeast Asia and afterward: An interview study of 898 Vietnam returnees. *Archives of General Psychiatry* **32**, 955–61.

Robins, L.N., Helzer, J.E., Hesselbrock, M. and Wish, E. (1980) Vietnam veterans three years after Vietnam: How our study changed our view of heroin. In: Brill, L. and Winick, C. (eds), *Yearbook of Substance Use and Abuse*, pp. 213–30. New York: Human Sciences Press.

Robson, P. (1998) Cannabis as a medicine; time for the phoenix to rise? *British Medical Journal* **316**, 1034–5.

Roe, S. and Man, L. (2006) *Drug Misuse Declared: Findings from the 2005/06 British Crime Survey*, (England and Wales), Home Office Statistical Bulletin 15/06, October. London: Home Office.

Roman, C.G., Ahn-Redding, H. and Simon, R.J. (2005) *Illicit Drug Policies, Trafficking, and Use the World Over*. Lanham, MD: Lexington Books.

Room, R. (1999) The rhetoric of international drug control. *Substance Use and Misuse* **34**, 1689–1707.

Room, R. (2005) Symbolism and rationality in the politics of psychoactive substances. In: Lindgren, B. and Grossman, M. (eds), *Substance Use: Individual Behavior, Social Interactions, Markets and Politics*, Advances in Health Economics and Health Services Research, vol. 16. Amsterdam: Elsevier, 331–46.

Room, R. (2005) Stigma, social inequality and alcohol and drug use. *Drug and Alcohol Review* **24**, 143–55.

Rosenberg, M. (1965) *Society and Adolescent Self-Image*. Princeton, NJ: Princeton University Press.

Roques, B. (1998) *La Dangerosité des Drogues - Rapport au Secrétariat d'Etat à la Santé*. Paris: Editions Odile Jacob La Documentation Française.

Royal College of General Practitioners (1986) *Alcohol: A Balanced View*. London: Tavistock.

Royal College of Physicians (1987) *Alcohol: A Great and Growing Evil: The Medical Consequences of Alcohol Abuse*. London: Tavistock.

Royal College of Physicians (2001a) *Alcohol-Can the NHS Afford it?* London: Royal College of Physicians.

Royal College of Physicians (2001b) *Nicotine Addiction in Britain*. London: Royal College of Physicians.

Royal College of Psychiatrists (1979) *Alcohol and Alcoholism*. London: Tavistock.

Royal College of Psychiatrists (1986) *Alcohol: Our Favourite Drug*. London: Tavistock.

Royal College of Psychiatrists (1987) *Drug Scenes*. London: Royal College of Psychiatrists.

Royal College of Psychiatrists (1988) Benzodiazepines and dependence: a College statement. *Bulletin of the Royal College of Psychiatrists* **12**, 107–8.

Royal Society of Arts Commission (2007) *Drugs–Facing the Facts*, March. London: Royal Society of Arts Commission.

Royal Society for the Encouragement of Arts, Manufactures and Commerce (2007) *Drugs-Facing Facts*. London: Royal Society for the Encouragement of Arts, Manufactures and Commerce, http://www.rsa.org.uk/projects/drugs.asp.

Royal United Services Institute for Defence and Security Studies (2007) British Army Loses 'Batallion' a Year to Drug-Use Discharges, December, http://www.rusi.org/news/ref:N47616079DFD16/

Rudat, K., Ryan, H. and Speed, M. (1992a) *Today's Young Adults: 16-19-Year-Olds Look at Diet, Alcohol, Drugs and Sexual Behaviour*. London: Health Education Authority.

Rudat, K., Speed, M. and Ryan, H. (1992b) *Tomorrow's Young Adults: 9-15-Year-Olds Look at Alcohol, Drugs, Exercise and Smoking*. London: Health Education Authority.

Ruddy, D. and Brown, A. (2007) *Experience of Drug Misuse: Findings from the 2006/07 Northern Ireland Crime Survey*. Belfast: Statistics and Research Branch, Northern Ireland Office.

Rudgley, R. (1995) The archaic use of hallucinogens in Europe: an archaeology of altered states. *Addiction* **90**, 163–4.

Rudgely, R. (1998) *The Alchemy of Cultures: Intoxicants in Society*. London: British Museum Press.

Rudgley, R. (2001) *Wildest Dreams: An Anthology of Drug –Related Literature*. London: Abacus.

Rumsfeld, D. (2002) *Statement made at Press Conference at NATO Headquarters*, 6 June. Brussels: NATO.

Samoirini, G. (2002) *Animals and Psychedelics: The Natural World and the Instinct to Alter Consciousness*. Rochester, VT: Park Street Press.

Schaps , E., Dibartolo, R., Moskowitz, J., Bailey, C.G. and Churgin, G. (1981) A review of 127 drug abuse prevention program evaluations. *Journal of Drug Issues* **11**, 17–43.

Schivelbusch, W. (1992) *Tastes of Paradise: A Social History of Intoxicants*. New York: Vintage Books.

Schlosser, E. (2004) *Reefer Madness: and other Tales from the American Underground*. Harmondsworth, Penguin.

Schofield, M. (1971) *The Strange Case of Pot*. Harmondsworth: Pelican.

Schulenberg, J.E. and Maggs, J.L. (2008) Destiny matters: distal developmental influences on adult use and abuse. *Addiction* **103**, 1–6.

Schultes, R.E. (1976) *Hallucinogenic Plants*. New York: Golden Press.

Schur, E.M. (1966) *Narcotic Addiction in Britain and America*. London: Tavistock.

Science and Technology Committee (2006) *Drug Classification*: *Making a Hash of it?*, 5th report. London: House of Commons.

Scotland's Futures Forum (2008) *Approaches to Alcohol and Drugs in Scotland: A Question of Architecture*, http://scotlandfutureforum.org/assets/files/report.pdf

Scott, P. and Willcox, D.R. (1965) Delinquency and amphetamines. *British Journal of Addiction* **61**, 9–27.

Scottish Government (2001) Cash boost and new targets for Scotland against Drugs, 19 February, http://www.scotland.gov.uk/News/Releases/2001/02/e1c0d17f-6140-4ca6-bd84-c6b3b15d2bd8

Scottish Government (2008) *The Road to Recovery: A New Approach to Tackling Scotland's Drug Problem*. Edinburgh: Scottish Government. http://www.scotland.gov.uk/Publications/2008/05/22161610/0

Scottish Government (2009) *Alcohol Bill*, http://www.scotland.gov.uk/About/programme-for-government/2009-10/summary-of-bills/alcohol-bill

Scottish Home and Health Department (1986) *HIV Infection in Scotland*, report of the Scottish Committee on HIV Infection and Intravenous Drug Misuse. Edinburgh: Scottish Home and Health Department.

Scottish Intercollegiate Guidelines Network (2007) *Management of Hepatitis C. A National Clinical Guideline.* Edinburgh: Scottish Intercollegiate Guidelines Network (SIGN).

Seaman, S.R., Brettle, R. and Gore, S.M. (1998) Mortality from overdose among injecting drug users recently released from prison: database linkage study. *British Medical Journal* **316**, 426–8.

Seddon, T. (2000) Explaining the Drug - Crime Link: Theoretical, Policy and Research Issues. *Journal of Social Policy* **29**, 95–107.

Senlis Council (2007) *Stumbling into Chaos: Afghanistan on the Brink.* London: M.F. Publishing.

Sense about Science (2009) *Principles for the Treatment of Independent Scientific Advice,* 6 November, http://www.senseaboutscience.org.uk/index.php/site/project/421

Shapiro, H. (ed.) (2008) *The Essential Student Reader on Drugs.* London: College Hill Press.

Shaw, A., Egan, J. and Gillespie, M. (2007) *Drugs and Poverty: A Literature Review.* Glasgow: Scottish Drugs Forum.

Shaw, C. and Bellis, M. (2009) Letter Introducing Report by Shaw al. 2009, 10 June.

Shaw, C., Hurst, A., McVeigh, J. and Bellis, M. (eds) (2009) *Indications of Public Health in the English Regions 10: Drug Use.* York: Association of Public Health Observatories.

Sherlock, K. (1999) Patterns of ecstasy use amongst club-goers on the UK dance scene. *International Journal of Drug Policy* **10**, 117–29.

Shewan, D. and Dalgarno, P. (2005) Low levels of negative health and social outcomes among non-treatment heroin users in Glasgow (Scotland): evidence for controlled heroin use?' *British Journal of Health Psychology* **10**, 1–17.

Shiman L.L. (undated) *Crusade against Drink in Victorian England.* London. MacMillan Press.

Simoens, S., Matheson, C., Inkster, K., Ludbrook, A. and Bond, C. (2002) *The Effectiveness of Treatment for Opiate Dependent Drug Users: An International Systematic Review of the Evidence,* Department of General Practice and Primary Care, and Health Economics Research Unit, University of Aberdeen, Scottish Executive Drug Misuse Research Programme, http://www.drugmisuse.isdscotland.org/eiu/pdfs/eiu_opi.pdf

Single, E., Robson, L., Xie, X. and Rehm, J. (1998) The economic costs of alcohol, tobacco and illicit drugs in Canada, 1992. *Addiction* **93**, 991–1006.

Singleton, N., Meltzer, H., Gatward, R., Cold, J. and Deasy, D. (1998) *Psychiatric Morbidity among Prisoners in England and Wales.* London: Office of National Statistics.

Singleton, N., Farrell, M. and Meltzer, H. (1999) *Substance Misuse among Prisoners in England and Wales.* London: Office for National Statistics.

Singleton, N., Pendry, E., Simpson, T., Goddard, E., Farrell, M., Marsden, J. and Taylor, C. (2005) *The Impact and Effectiveness of Mandatory Drug Testing in Prisons,* Findings 223. London: Home Office.

Skidmore, C.A., Robertson, J.R., Robertson, A.A. and Elton, R.A. (1990) After the epidemic: follow up study of HIV seroprevalence and changing patterns of drug use. *British Medical Journal* **300**, 219–23.

Sky News (2009) Drugs behind many arrests of Britons abroad, 25 August, http://news.sky.com/skynews/Home/UK-News/Drug-Offences-Account-For-Many-Arrests-Of-

Britons-Abroad-Says-Foreign-And-Commonwealth-Office/
Article/200908415367820?f=rss

Slack, J. and Brogan, B. (2008) Cannabis: At last a U-turn. *Daily Mail* 29 April, pp. 1, 4.

Small, D. and Drucker, E. (2008) Return to Galileo? The inquisition of the International Narcotics Control Board. *Harm Reduction Journal* **5**, 16

Smart, R.G. and Ogborne, A.C. (2000) Drug use and drinking among students in 36 countries. *Addictive Behaviors* **25**, 455–60.

Smith, C. and Nutbeam, D. (1992) Adolescent drug use in Wales. *British Journal of Addiction* **87**, 227–33.

Smith, T.W. (1995) Trends in non-response rates. *International Journal of Public Opinion Research* **7**, 157–71.

Smout, T.C. and Wood, S. (1991) *Scottish voices 1745-1960.* London: Fontana Press.

Sneader, W. (2005) *Drug Discovery.* London: Wiley.

Solowij, N., Hall, W. and Lee, N. (2006) Recreational MDMA use in Sydney: A profile of 'ecstasy' users and their experiences with the drug. *Addiction* **87**, 1161–72.

South, N. (ed.) (1999) *Drugs: Cultures, Controls and Everyday Life.* London: Sage.

Spender Q. (2004) Assessment of adolescent self harm. *Current Paediatrics* **15**, 2: 120–6.

Squires, N.F., Beeching, N.J., Schlecht, B.J. and Ruben, S.M. (1995) An estimate of the prevalence of drug misuse in Liverpool and a spatial analysis of known addiction. *Journal of Public Health Medicine* **17**, 103–9.

Standage, T. (2005) *A History of the World in Six Glasses.* London: Atlantic Books.

Stanton, B., Li, X., Galbraith, J., Cornick, G., Feigelman, S., Kaljee, L. and Zhou, Y. (2000) Parental underestimates of adolescent risk behavior: a randomized, controlled trial of a parental monitoring intervention. *Journal of Adolescent Health* **26**, 18–26.

Steele, J. (2007) Police chiefs u-turn on cannabis classification. *Daily Telegraph* 21 November, http://www.telegraph.co.uk/news/main.jhtml?xml=/news/2007/11/21/ncannabis121.xml

Stewart, K. and Sweedler, B.M. (1997) Driving under the influence. In: Plant, M.A., Single, E. and Stockwell, T. (eds), *Alcohol: Minimising the Harm: What Works?*, pp. 126–42. London: Free Association Books.

Stimson, G.V. (1973) *Heroin and Behaviour.* Shannon: Irish University Press.

Stimson, G.V. and Oppenheimer, E. (1982) *Heroin Addiction.* London: Tavistock.

Strang, J. and Stimson, G.V. (eds) (1990) *AIDS and Drug Misuse.* London: Tavistock/ Routeledge.

Stringer, C. (2006) *Homo Britannicus: The Incredible Story of Human Life in Britain.* Harmondsworth: Penguin.

Stringer, C. and Andrews, P. (2005) *The Complete World of Human Evolution.* London: Thames and Hudson.

Stockwell, T., Gruenewald., P.J., Toumbourou, J.W. and Loxley, W. (eds) (2005) *Preventing Harmful Substance Abuse.* Chichester: Wiley.

Substance Abuse and Mental Health Services Administration (2005) Characteristics of primary admissions by age of first use of alcohol: 2002, 14 April, http://www.oas.samhsa.gov/2k5/alcAgeTX/alcAgeTX.htm

Sullivan, R.J. and Hagen, H. (2002) Psychotropic substance-seeking: evolutionary pathology or adaptation? *Addiction* **97**, 389–400.

Sumnall, H.R., Tyler, E., Wagstaff, G.F. and Cole, J.C. (2004) A behavioural economic analysis of alcohol, amphetamine, cocaine and ecstasy purchases by polydrug users. *Drug and Alcohol Dependence* **76**, 93–9.

Sutton, M. and Maynard, A. (1992) *What is the Size and Nature of the 'drug' problem in the UK?*, YARTIC Occasional Paper 3. York: Centre for Health Economics, University of York.

Swadi, H. (1988) Drug and substance use among 3,333 London adolescents. *British Journal of Addiction* **83**, 935–42.

Swadi, H. (1999) Individual risk factors for adolescent substance use. *Drug and Alcohol Dependence* **55**, 209–24.

Syal, R. (2009) Drug money 'saved the banks' in global crisis. *The Observer* 13 December, p. 4.

Symonds, J. (1973) *The Great Beast: The Life and Magick of Aleister Crowley*. London: Mayflower.

The National Center on Addiction and Substance Abuse at Columbia University (CASA) (2007) *National Survey of American Attitudes on Substance Abuse XII: Teens and Parents*. New York, CASA.

The Guardian (2000) *Guardian/ICM poll on attitudes to drug law*. 17 October.

The Observer (2008) Mushrooms move. *The Observer* 27 April, p. 8.

Thompson, T. (2007) *Reefer Men*. London: Hodder and Stoughton.

Thorley A: (1981) Longitudinal studies of drug dependence. In: Edwards, G. and Busch, C. (eds), *Drug Problems in Britain: A Review of Ten Years*, pp. 117–69. London: Academic Press.

Thornton, S. (1996) *Club Cultures: Music, Media and Subcultural Capital, Middletown*. Connecticut: Wesleyan University Press.

Times Online (2007) Outcry after UNICEF identifies UK's 'failed generation' of children, 14 February, http://www.timesonline.co.uk/tol/news/world/europe/article1384238.ece

Tisdall, S. and MacAskill, E. (2006) America's long war. *The Guardian* 15 February, p. 19.

Tobler, N. (1986) Meta-analysis of 143 adolescent drug abuse prevention programs: Quantitative results of program participants compared to a control or comparison group. *Journal of Drug Issues* **16**, 537–67.

Todd, J., Currie, C. and Smith, R. (1999) *Health Behaviours of Scottish schoolchildren, Technical Report 1: Smoking, Drinking and Drug Use in the 1990s*. Edinburgh: Research Unit in Health & Behaviour Change, The University of Edinburgh.

Travis, A. (2007) Fewer young people using cannabis after reclassification. *The Guardian* 25 October, http://www.guardian.co.uk/drugs/Story/0,2198881,00.html

Travis, A. (2009a) Younger cocaine users more at risk from adulterated drugs. *The Guardian* 10 June, p. 9.

Travis, A. (2009b) Revealed: the hidden army in UK prisons. *The Guardian* 25 September, p. 1.

Trocchi, A. (1960) *Cain's Book*. London: Calder.

Tyler, A. (1986) *Street Drugs*. London: New English Library.

Tyrer, P. (1987) Benefits and risks of benzodiazepines. In: Freeman, H. and Rue, Y. (eds), *The Benzodiazepines in Current Clinical Practice*, pp. 3–11. London: Royal Society of Medicine Services.

UK Drug Policy Commission (2007) *An Analysis of UK Drug Policy*, P. Reuter and A. Stevens, www.ukdpc.org.uk

UK Drug Policy Commission (2008) *Reducing Drug Use, Reducing Reoffending: are Programmes for Problem Drug-using Offenders in the UK Supported by the Evidence?* London: UK Drug Policy Commission.

United Nations (1961) *United Nations Single Convention on Narcotic Drugs.* New York: United Nations.

United Nations (1971) *United Nations Convention on Psychotropic Drugs.* New York: United Nations.

United Nations (1988) *United Nations Convention against Illicit Traffic in Narcotic Drugs and Psychotropic Substances.* New York: United Nations.

United Nations (2009) *World Drug Report*, pp. 23–245. New York: United Nations Office on Drugs and Crime (UNODC).

United Nations Childrens' Fund (UNICEF) (2007) *An Overview of Child Well-Being in Rich Countries: A Comprehensive Assessment of the Lives and Well-being of Children and Adolescents in the Economically Advanced Nations*, Report Card 7, http://www.unicef irc.org//presscentre/presskit/reportcard7/rc7_eng.pd

United Nations Development Program (2006) *Human Development Report.* New York: Oxford University Press.

United Nations News Centre (2008) *Opium Cultivation in Afghanistan drops by a Fifth, Finds UN Survey*, 26 August, http://www.un.org/apps/news/story.asp?NewsID=27819 &Cr=afghan&Cr1=drug

United Nations Office on Drugs and Crime (2005) *World Drug Report 2005.* Vienna: United Nations Office on Drugs and Crime.

United Nations Office on Drugs and Crime (2008) *World Drug Report 2008*, http://www. unodc.org/documents/wdr/WDR_2008/WDR_2008_eng_web.pdf

United Nations Office on Drugs and Crime (2009a) *World Drug Report 2009*, http://www. unodc.org/unodc/en/data-and-analysis/WDR-2009.html

United Nations Office on Drugs and Crime (2009b) *Afghan Opium Survey*. Vienna: United Nations Office on Drugs and Crime, http://www.unodc.org/unodc/en/drugs/afghan-opium-survey.html

Van Asten, L.C., Boufassa, F., Schiffer, V., Brettle, R.P., Robertson, J.R., Hernandez Aguado, I., McMenamin, J., Zangerle, R., Fontanet, A. et al. (2003a) Limited effect of highly active antiretroviral therapy among HIV-positive injecting drug users on the population level. *European Journal of Public Health* **13**, 347–9.

Van Asten, L., Langendam, M., Zangerle, R., Hernandez Aguado, I., Boufassa, F., Schiffer, V., Brettle, R.P., Robertson, J.R., Fontanet, A., Coutinho, R.A. and Prins, M. (2003b) Tuberculosis risk varies with the duration of HIV infection: a prospective study of European drug users with known date of HIV seroconversion. *AIDS* **17**, 1201–8.

Van Asten, L., Verhaest, I., Lamzira, S., Hernandez-Aguado, I., Zangerle, R., Boufassa, F., Rezza, G., Broers, B., Robertson, J.R., Brettle, R.P. et al. (2004) European and Italian Seroconverter Studies. Spread of hepatitis C virus among European injection drug users infected with HIV: a phylogenetic analysis. *Journal of Infectious Diseases* **189**, 292–302.

Van Der Vorst, H., Engels, R.C.M.E., Meeus, W., Deković, M and Van Leeuwe, J. (2005a) The role of alcohol specific socialization on adolescents' drinking behaviour. *Addiction* **100**, 1464–74.

Van Der Vorst, H., Engels, R.C.M.E., Meeus, W. and Deković, M. (2005b) The impact of rules, parental norms and parental alcohol use on adolescent drinking behaviour. *Journal of Child Psychology and Psychiatry* 47, 1299–1306.

Van Der Vorst, H., Engels, R.C.M.E., Meeus, W. and Deković, M. (2006) Parental attachment, parental control and early development of alcohol use: a longitudinal study. *Psychology of Addictive Behavior* 20, 107–16.

Vastag, B. (2003) GAO: DARE does not work. *Journal of the American Medical Association* 289, 539.

Velleman, R. (2009) *Influences on How Children and Young People Learn about and Behave towards Alcohol.* York: Joseph Rowntree Foundation.

Velleman, R. and Orford, J. (1999) *Risk and Resilience: Adults who were the Children of Problem Drinkers.* Amsterdam: Harwood Academic Publishers.

Velleman, R. and Templeton, L. (2003) Alcohol, drugs and the family: Results from a long-running research program within the UK. *European Addiction Research* 9, 103–12.

Velleman, R., Copello, A. and Maslin, J. (eds) (1998) *Living with Drink.* London: Longman.

Vivancos, R., Maskrey, V., Rumball, D., Harvey, I. and Holland, R. (2006) Crack/cocaine use in a rural county of England. *Journal of Public Health* 2, 96–103.

Waldorf, D. (1973) *Careers in Dope.* Englewod Cliffs, NJ: Prentice Hall.

Walsh, I. (1996) *Trainspotting.* New York: W.W. Norton & Company.

Warburton, D.M. (1988) The puzzle of nicotine use. In: Lader, M. (ed.), *The Psychopharmacology of Addiction*, pp. 27–49. Oxford: Oxford University Press.

Warner, J. (2003) *Craze: Gin and Debauchery in an Age of Reason.* London: Profile.

Watts, J. (2009) Western Eye drugs survey: The results. *Western Eye* (University of the West of England, Bristol student newspaper), 7, 6–7.

Webb, E., Ashton, C.H., Kelly, P. and Kamali, F. (1996) Alcohol and drug use in UK university students. *Lancet* 348, 9232–9925.

Weisheit, R. (1983) The social context of alcohol and drug education: Implications for program evaluations. *Journal of Alcohol & Drug Education* 2, 72–81.

Weitoft, G., Hjern, A., Haglund, B. and Rosén, M. (2003) Mortality, severe morbidity, and injury in children living with single parents in Sweden: a population-based study. *Lancet* 361, 289–95.

Welsh Assembly Government (2008) *Working Together to Reduce Harm.* Cardiff: Welsh Assembly Government.

Welsh Assembly Government (2008) *New 10 Year Plan to Reduce the Harm Caused by Drugs and Alcohol* (press release), 1 October, http://wales.gov.uk/news/topic/health/2008/081001plan/?lang=en

Welsh Office (1996) *Forward Together: A Strategy to Combat Drug and Alcohol Misuse in Wales.* Cardiff: The Welsh Office.

West, R. and Hardy, A. (2006) *Theory of Addiction.* Oxford: Blackwell.

Westwood, J. and Mullen, B. (2009) Young people and sexual risk taking behavior in Central England. *Sexual Health* 6, 135–8.

Whitaker et al. (2000)Whitaker, D.J. and Miller, K.S. (2000) Parent-Adolescent Discussions about Sex and Condoms: Impact on Peer Influences of Sexual Risk Behavior. *Journal of Adolescent Research* 15, 251–73.

Wickström, P.-O. and Butterworth, D.A. (2007) *Adolescent Crime*. Uffculme, Devon: Willan Publishing.

Wiederman M.W. and Pryor T. (1996) Substance use and impulsive behaviours among adolescents with eating disorders. *Addictive Behaviours* **21**, 269–72.

Wiener, R.S.P. (1970) *Drugs and Schoolchildren*. London: Longman.

Wiessing, L., Van de Laar, M.J., Donoghoe, M.C., Guarita, B., Klempová, D. and Griffiths, P. (2008) HIV among injecting drug users in Europe: Increasing trends in the East. *Surveillance* **50**, 11 December 2008.

Wilkinson, H. (1994) *No Turning Back: Generations and the Genderquake*. London: Demos.

Wilkinson, R.G. (2001) *Unhealthy Societies. The Afflictions of Inequality*. London: Routledge.

Wilkinson, R. and Picket, K. (2009) *The Spirit Level; Why Equality is Better for Everyone*. London: Penguin Books.

Williams, B. Chang, K. and Van Truong, M. (1992) *Canadian Profile: Alcohol and Other Drugs 1992*. Toronto, Addiction Research Foundation.

Williams, M. (1986) The Thatcher generation. *New Society* 21 February, pp. 312–15.

Williams, S., Hickman, M., Bottle, A. and Aylin, P. (2005) Hospital admissions for drug and alcohol use in people aged under 45. *British Medical Journal* **330**, 115.

Wilson, C.W.M. (ed.) (1968) *Adolescent Drug Use*. London: Pergamon.

Winehouse, A. (2006) Lyrics from "Rehab. *Back to Back*: Universal Republic Records.

Wodak A. (1998) Medical complications of drug use. In: Robertson, J.R. (ed.), *Management of Drug Users in the Community*. London: Arnold.

Wodak, A. and Lurie, P. (1996) A tale of two countries: attempts to control HIV among injecting drug users in Australia and the United States. *Journal of Drug Issues* **6**, 117–34.

Wodak, A., Fisher, R. and Crofts, N. (1993) An evolving public health crisis: HIV infection among injecting drug users in developing countries. In: Heather, N., Wodak, A., Nadelmann, E. and O'Hare, P. (eds), *Psychoactive Drugs and Harm Reduction from Faith to Science*, pp. 280–97. London: Whurr.

Wood, A.J. (1967) *Drug Dependence*. Bristol: Bristol Corporation and the British Council of Social Services.

Wood, M.D., Read, J., Mitchell, R.E. and Brand, N.H. (2004) Do parents matter? Parent and peer influences on alcohol involvement among recent high school graduates. *Psychology of Addictive Behavior* **18**, 19–30.

Wooding, D. (2009) Cabinet in drug war over sacking of Professor Nutt. *The Sun* 3 November, http://www.thesun.co.uk/sol/homepage/news/2711166/Cabinet-in-drug-war-over-sacking-of-Professor-David-Nutt.html

Woods, J.H., Katz, J.L. and Winger, G. (1992) Benzodiazepines: use, abuse and consequences. *Pharmacological Reviews* **44**, 151–338.

World Health Organization (1994) *International Classification of Diseases*. Geneva: World Health Organization.

World Health Organization (2002) *Mental Health and Substance Abuse*, 18 September, http://www.afro.who.int/mentalhealth/related_diseases/substance_abuse.html

World Health Organization (2004) *Global Status Report on Alcohol*. Geneva: World Health Organization.

Wright, J.D. and Pearl, L. (1995) Knowledge and experience of young people regarding drug misuse 1969-94, *British Medical Journal* **309**, 20–4.

Wylie, A.S., Scott, R.T. and Burnett, S.J. (1995) Psychosis due to 'skunk'. *British Medical Journal* **311**, 125.

York, J.L., Welte, J., Hirsch, J., Hoffman, J.H. and Barnes, G. (2004) Association of age of first drink with current alcohol drinking variables in a national general population sample. *Alcoholism: Clinical and Experimental Research* 28, 1379–87.

Young, J. (1971) *The Drugtakers*. London: Paladin.

Young, J. and Brooke Crutchley, J. (1972) Student drug use. *Drugs and Society* **1**, 11–15.

Zacune, J. and Hensman, C. (1971) *Drugs, Alcohol and Tobacco in Britain*. London: Heinemann.

Zigmond, A.S. and Snaith, R.P. (1983) The Hospital Anxiety and Depression Scale. *Acta Psychiatica Scandanavica* **67**, 361–70.

Zinberg, N.E. (1984) *Drug, Set and Setting: The Basis for Controlled Intoxicant Use*. New Haven, CT: Yale University Press.

Zucker, R.A. (2008) Anticipating problem alcohol use developmentally from childhood into middle adulthood: what have we learned? *Addiction* **103**, 100–9.

Index

Page numbers in *italic* indicate figures and tables.